From Wine Mom to Sober Mom

Alcohol Addiction and Recovery: A Story of Hope for Women

Howard Kane

Hidden Alpha Capital LLC

1st edition in 2025

About Author

HOWARD KANE WRITES THE stories most people are afraid to tell.

As a former Fortune 500 executive, he knows what it feels like to look successful on the outside while quietly unraveling on the inside. For years, he hid his drinking behind late nights, busy calendars, and a polished smile. When he finally faced the truth about his addiction, he discovered that recovery wasn't just possible. It was life-changing.

Howard channels that experience into powerful, memoir-style novels that expose the hidden cost of alcohol dependence and the courage it takes to break free. His first book, ***The Double Life of a High-Functioning Alcoholic***, pulls back the curtain on addiction that hides behind ambition and success. His second, ***From Wine Mommy to Sober Mommy***, shines a light on the unique struggles mothers face when alcohol threatens everything they love.

Through raw honesty and lived perspective, Howard's books reveal that sobriety isn't about getting life back. It's about building a stronger, truer one. Readers call his stories "impossible to put down" because they are as real as the people living them.

If you've ever questioned your relationship with drinking, Howard Kane's work offers both recognition and hope.

Website: https://selfcarejourneybooks.com/

Contents

Chapter One

The Knock

KNOCK. KNOCK. KNOCK.

The knock hit like thunder in the silence.

Sharp. Firm. The kind that doesn't ask for permission. It just landed, hard, like someone had dropped a weight on the quiet. My chest clenched before I even knew why.

I sat bolt upright on the couch. My neck screamed from the way I'd been slouched, half-passed out in front of some show I wasn't even watching. The kind you put on just to drown out the quiet. The takeout box from dinner lay tipped on the floor, lo mein noodles and sauce oozing across the hardwood like a greasy confession.

Knock. Knock. Knock.

"Police. We need to speak with Emily Matthews."

I froze. It took a second for the words to sink in. Then panic hit, sharp and sudden. Police. At my door. My eyes flicked to the cable box. Nine o'clock. I was still in my wine haze, and nothing was cleaned up. Not the dinner. Not the living room. Not me.

Then my brain clicked into people-pleasing mode. Appear normal. Look functional. Be the kind of mother who's got everything handled. Not the one who'd just drained an entire bottle of Pinot Grigio watching baking show reruns because the house felt too empty and I couldn't stand being in my own head.

I stood up too fast and almost stepped into the noodles. My shirt was wrinkled, sagging, with big block letters across the front: World's Best Mom. Emma gave it to me last year. I used to wear it on purpose. Tonight, it felt like a cruel joke waiting to show its punchline.

The hallway stretched ahead like part of a dream. My legs didn't feel attached to the ground. I put one hand on the wall to steady myself and tried to smooth my hair with the other.

Just breathe, Emily. Just breathe... You can handle this. You've talked your way out of worse situations.

Except I couldn't think of any worse situations.

I opened the door.

Two officers stood there, one older, one younger. The door light threw a hard glow across their faces. The older one had kind eyes, or maybe they were just tired. His name tag said Dalton. The younger one was already scribbling in a notepad, not even looking up.

"Ma'am, we received a welfare check request for this address. Are you Emily Matthews?"

"Yes." My voice cracked. I cleared my throat. "Yes, I'm Emily. Is something wrong?"

Even as I said it, I knew. I knew who called. I knew why.

"We need to check on the welfare of two minor children, Emma and Lucas Matthews. Are they here with you tonight?"

The hallway tilted just a little. I caught myself on the doorframe.

"Of course they're here. They just went to sleep. It's a school night."

I tried to sound offended, like the kind of mother who'd be outraged at the question. I could hear the edge in my voice, but they didn't buy it.

Dalton gave a small nod, but his eyes flicked to his partner. Something passed between them.

"Ma'am, we're going to need to see the children."

"You want to wake them up?" My stomach turned. "They just went to bed. They need their sleep."

"We just need to verify they're safe and well cared for," the younger one said. His voice was flat, his pen still moving.

I wanted to say no. Slam the door. Demand a warrant. Stand on my rights as a mother. But none of it would matter. They were going to see my kids, one way or another.

"Fine," I said. "But please be quiet. If they wake up, they'll be cranky tomorrow."

As if that was my biggest worry.

They stepped inside, and I saw my home through their eyes. Not in the half-light of denial, but as it really was. The wine glass on the floor. The bottle on the kitchen counter. Another bottle poking from the recycling bin. The stale air, like no one had opened a window in days. Emma's art project spread across the dining table. Lucas's toy trucks scattered in the hallway. Dishes from two, maybe three days ago.

"Please follow me," I said quietly, leading them to the kids' rooms. Every step felt heavier.

Emma's room was first. I opened the door slowly and carefully. She was curled under her unicorn blanket, her little chest rising and falling with each breath. Her blonde hair fanned across the pillow like something out of a shampoo ad. A book lay open beside her. She must have fallen asleep reading. Her cheeks were flushed. She looked peaceful.

Dalton leaned in. "She looks good," he said softly.

Of course she did. Whatever else I'd done wrong, I hadn't let anything happen to them. Not yet. That was still my line, the one thing I hadn't crossed.

Lucas's room was next. Four years old, tiny. Tangled in his dinosaur blanket, half-hanging off the bed, his stuffed dinosaur clutched in one hand. Toy trucks scattered across the mattress. He must have fallen asleep mid-play. His breathing was deep and steady.

"Both children appear healthy and safe," Dalton said to his partner, who kept writing like none of this was new.

We went back to the living room in silence. My bare feet felt every crumb and dent in the floor. The takeout on the floor seemed to glow under the lamp now, waiting to betray me.

Dalton looked at me. His tone shifted, colder.

"Ma'am, we can smell alcohol. Have you been drinking tonight?"

The lie was ready. I'd used it a hundred times. Just one glass. Just dinner. Just normal. But I couldn't get it out.

"I had some wine," I said. "After the kids went to bed."

"How much?" the younger one asked.

How much? Like there was a number that made it okay. Like one glass would make them nod and leave. But they'd seen the bottle. They'd smelled it on me.

"I don't know," I said. "A normal amount."

They stayed another twenty minutes. Asked about my job. I still had one, barely. Asked about childcare. My mom helped when she could. Asked about my support system. I didn't have one. Asked if I thought I had a drinking problem. I told them no. Everyone drinks wine.

Dalton handed me a card with numbers for social services. The other one said they'd be filing a report. Words like follow-up, caseworker, and child safety landed like matches on dry leaves.

When they left, I locked the door and leaned against it. I waited until I heard their car pull away, then just stood there. Everything was still. Too still.

I stared at the wine glass on the floor. At the sticky noodles. At my shirt. At the life I'd been pretending was still under control.

I went back to see my kids again. I needed to see them one more time, just to make sure.

Emma hadn't moved. Still tucked into her blanket, clutching her bunny. Lucas was wrapped up like a little burrito. They were safe. Still mine. For now.

I kissed their foreheads. I whispered I loved them. And I meant it.

Then I went into the bathroom and turned on the light.

The mirror didn't lie. It never had. I just stopped looking.

A woman stared back with bloodshot eyes and hollow cheeks. Her skin looked gray. Her shirt was stained. Her hair hung limp. But it was the eyes that stopped me. They belonged to someone else. Someone who had given up. Someone who drank wine at noon and called it brunch. Someone who broke promises to her kids and still swore she was a good mother.

Someone whose ex had to call the police to check if her kids were safe.

I gripped the counter until my knuckles went white.

This was the moment. Not the night Jake left. Not the day I lost the promotion. Not the morning I forgot Emma's lunch.

This was the moment I had to decide if I was going to keep pretending I was fine, or finally admit I wasn't.

It was 10:15.

In the morning, my kids would ask for breakfast. Cereal. Help tying their shoes. They would look at me like I had all the answers.

I splashed cold water on my face.

The woman in the mirror still looked like a mess. But she was still their mom.

Maybe that was enough. Maybe it was the first step.

The mess on the floor could wait.

There were bigger things to clean up.

And after tonight, everything had to change.

Chapter Two

Freshman Year Freedom

I STOOD IN THE bathroom that night, clutching the sink, staring at the person in the mirror. My face looked gray under the harsh light. Eyes bloodshot, skin dull, the t-shirt clinging to me like a joke I didn't get anymore. The silence in the house felt different now. Not peaceful. Not private. Just exposed.

And I kept asking myself the same question. How did I get here?

How did a woman who once graduated magna cum laude, who had a full scholarship, a plan, a future, end up like this? So far gone that her ex-husband had to call the police to check on her kids?

I used to think the turning point was the first blackout. Or the first time I lied about how much I drank. Or the night the custody fight started, when I realized just how thin the ground beneath me had become.

But the truth was harder. It went deeper.

It started long before I knew there was something to lose. Back in a time and place that now feels almost imaginary. A different life. A different version of me.

It started when drinking still felt like freedom.

The back window of my parents' Honda shrank until it disappeared around the dorm parking lot corner. And just like that, my childhood was gone.

I stood there on the sidewalk, milk crates of my life stacked around me, watching the emptiness settle in. I was eighteen, fresh out of high school with a full ride to a prestigious university. Straight-A student, debate team captain, valedictorian. And for the first time in my life, nobody was watching.

The air was thick with possibility. And fear. But mostly freedom.

"You must be Emily!" someone chirped behind me.

I turned to see a girl with impossibly shiny hair and a pageant-winner smile. "I'm Jessica, your resident assistant. Ready for the best four years of your life?"

I smiled back, polite, unsure. I didn't know then just how right she was. Or how wrong.

That first week was a blur of awkward icebreakers, mystery meat at the dining hall, and the jarring intimacy of sharing a shoebox-sized dorm room with someone I'd never met. My roommate Katie was a farm girl from Nebraska who brought an actual quilt her grandma made and printed photos of her dog and baby cousins. It felt like she was trying to transplant her whole life onto the cinderblock walls.

I unpacked my laptop, textbooks, and a case of energy drinks I'd convinced myself were crucial for academic survival. I thought I was being practical. Looking back, I was just trying to hold on to control.

The first party came three days in.

"Come on, Emily," Katie begged, standing in front of the mirror with a lip gloss in hand like she was prepping for surgery. "It's just a mixer for the honors dorm. How wild could it possibly be?"

Those are the kind of words that always lead to trouble.

The party was in the basement of Wellington Hall, lit by cheap string lights and filled with nervous overachievers pretending to be chill. The punch was bright red and definitely spiked, though no one said it out loud. Everyone stood in awkward little circles, trying too hard not to try too hard.

That's when Madison from my calculus class handed me a bottle.

"It's just a wine cooler," she said, like she was offering me a juice box. "My mom lets me have them at home."

I hesitated for half a second before taking it, the condensation slick against my fingers. The bottle was cold and sticky, its label peeling at the edges. I twisted the cap off, surprised at how easily it gave way, like it had been waiting for me.

The first sip was sweeter than I expected. Syrupy, like melted Jolly Ranchers. Artificial fruit with a bite of something sharp underneath. It didn't taste like alcohol the way I'd imagined. It tasted like a secret. Like something I wasn't supposed to like but did anyway.

I tried to play it cool, holding the bottle like I'd done this before, nodding along to the music in the background, even though my hand trembled just enough that I had to switch it to the other. My whole body felt suddenly electric, like someone had turned the volume up on my skin.

Each sip made the world shift a little. The noise in the room stopped scraping at me. My shoulders dropped. My breath became easier. The tight coil of worry I always carried (the pressure to be good, to be perfect, to never mess up) unwound just enough for me to forget it was there.

By the time I finished, the colors around me felt warmer. Softer. The edges had blurred just enough to stop cutting. The music seemed to pour into me instead of bouncing off. And I caught myself laughing, really laughing, without first checking who was watching.

I didn't feel afraid. I didn't feel small. I just felt... light.

And that feeling (that buzz under my skin, that sudden sense that maybe I was enough without trying so hard) was the part I wanted more of.

That was it. The moment I started believing alcohol could fix things.

In October, I rushed to a sorority. And that's when drinking stopped being cute.

"Alright, ladies," Brittany barked, standing on a couch in the Kappa basement in ripped jeans and the confidence of someone who ruled the world. "Tonight, we're gonna teach you how to party like a Kappa."

The room had been transformed into an alcohol obstacle course. Beer pong in one corner, flip cup in another, a table for "power hour," which meant taking a shot of beer every single minute for sixty minutes straight.

"The key is to know your limits," Brittany grinned, "and then push past them."

I'd always been competitive. I didn't know how not to be. So, I tackled drinking the same way I'd tackled AP exams and speech tournaments. I wanted to win.

And I did. I was good at it.

By Halloween, I had a rhythm. Wine coolers during study sessions. Beer at parties. Vodka when I needed courage. It wasn't about getting wasted. It was about becoming someone else.

The girl who walked into parties like she'd always been there. Who laughed easily and didn't overthink every word. Who flirted without anxiety and made friends without trying. The girl who felt light. Effortless. Fun.

At night, while Katie spread her chem books across our shared desk, I'd pour a glass from the bottle I kept tucked behind my sweaters. Just enough to blur the edges. To make everything feel less serious. Less sharp.

"Doesn't that make it harder to study?" Katie asked once, eyeing me as I highlighted a chapter in my psych textbook.

"No, it helps me focus," I said, and I meant it. That buzz made everything easier. "My dad has a glass of wine every night with the paper. It's what adults do."

Katie blinked like she didn't quite know what to say. She was pre-med, with a five-year plan and a high school sweetheart waiting back home. She didn't need wine to feel steady.

I envied her for that. And I pitied her for it too.

Spring semester was when Jake Matthews came into the picture. And with him came a new kind of drinking. The kind that didn't just take the edge off or make me feel confident. It made everything feel romantic.

I first noticed him at Murphy's Pub, that off-campus dive with greasy burgers and bartenders who didn't ask too many questions. He was sitting with a bunch of business school guys, laughing at something, leaning back like the world belonged to him. It wasn't just a smile. It was the way he listened when other people talked. The way he held his beer like it was no big deal, like drinking wasn't about nerves or pressure. Just something normal people did.

"Excuse me," he said later, appearing next to me at the bar. "You're in Professor Wilson's macro class, right? I'm Jake Matthews."

"Emily," I said. I could actually meet his eyes, thanks to the two beers already in my system. "You sit three rows behind me."

"I do," he said, smiling again. "Can I buy you a drink?"

That one drink turned into three. Then into two hours of leaning in too close, sharing stories about everything and nothing. He told me he was majoring in econ, wanted to work in finance, and when he talked about the stock market, his whole face lit up. Like it wasn't about money. Like it was magic.

When I told him I was studying communications, he asked real questions. Not the polite kind. He actually listened.

Eventually, I glanced at the time and realized it was past midnight. "I should probably head back."

"Let me walk you," he said, already reaching for his wallet and dropping cash on the bar without a second thought.

The walk back to my dorm felt unreal. We were both tipsy and young, wrapped up in that soft buzz where everything felt like a movie. He told me about growing up in Connecticut, wanting to move to New York, and some summer trip to Europe he was planning. He spoke like someone who had already figured it all out.

"What about you?" he asked when we reached my building. "What's your five-year plan?"

I laughed, not because I had an answer, but because I didn't. "I guess I'm still figuring that out."

"I like that," he said. "Keeps things interesting."

When he kissed me goodnight, I tasted beer and hope... that dangerous feeling that maybe, just maybe, this could turn into something real.

Our first official date was at Romano's, the nicest restaurant within walking distance of campus. Jake ordered a bottle of wine with confidence that made it feel like we belonged there. He swirled it in the glass like he'd seen in movies and handed it to me with a grin.

"To new beginnings," he said.

"To new beginnings," I echoed, pretending I was just as grown-up as he looked.

The wine was smoother than anything I'd ever tasted. Rich. Expensive. He talked about internship interviews while I twirled pasta around my fork and soaked in every second. For a moment, I felt like the version of myself I always imagined I'd become. Smart. Attractive. In control. The kind of girl who could handle a relationship and a bottle of wine at the same time.

By spring break, we were officially together. And drinking had woven itself so tightly into my life that I barely noticed it anymore. It was just part of the rhythm.

We went to Panama City Beach with a group of friends and checked into a motel that smelled like chlorine, beer, and bad choices. The plan was simple. Drinking on the beach all day. Club-hopping all night. Waking up somewhere in between.

"Shots!" my sorority sister Melissa yelled on the first night, carrying a tray of something blue and neon. "Spring break rules. No counting. No limits. No regrets."

I hadn't done shots before. But Jake handed me one with a wink.

"When in Rome," he said.

The burn was awful. But the warmth afterward? That part was familiar. And welcome. One shot turned into three. Then five. Then the number stopped mattering. At some point I ended up dancing on a table while Jake stood below cheering me on, laughing like this was the most fun anyone could ever have.

The next morning, I woke up on the bathroom floor. My head throbbed. My stomach flipped. I was wearing someone else's bikini top and had no idea how I got there.

"Rough night?" Jake said, stepping over a pile of towels and seeing me slumped against the toilet. He looked half-concerned, half-amused. Like this was a rite of passage.

"I think I overdid it," I muttered, rubbing my temples.

"Welcome to spring break," he said, then offered me a beer like it was breakfast. "Hair of the dog?"

I hesitated, then took it. That was just what you did. You didn't sit around sulking while everyone else had fun. You drank through it. Laughed it off. Got back in the game.

That beer led to another. Then another. We drank on the sand all day, danced at clubs all night, and the whole trip blurred into this loud, sunburned, half-remembered haze. By the time we made it back to campus, I'd had my first blackout. My first real hangover didn't fade after a nap. My first whisper of doubt, wondering if maybe I'd taken things too far.

But no one else seemed to think so. Jake thought it was hilarious. My sorority sisters called me a legend. The blurry photos from that week made it into our group chat with laughing emojis and captions like "never forget."

I was fitting in. Better than ever.

Senior year came faster than I was ready for. One minute I was figuring out my class schedule for junior fall, and the next I was updating my resume, obsessing over job interviews, and filling out grad school applications. The pressure was relentless. What was I going to do next? Where would I go? Who would I be?

Still, my grades were solid. More than solid. I'd kept my scholarship, kept up appearances, kept everything looking sharp from the outside. My social life seemed full and normal. I had friends. I had Jake. I had it together.

The glass of wine I used to pour while studying had quietly turned into two. Sometimes three, especially on nights when Jake was out with his frat brothers and I was alone in my apartment, trying to pretend the silence didn't feel so heavy.

By junior year, I'd moved off-campus into a little one-bedroom that felt like luxury compared to dorm life. I had hardwood floors, and actual glassware. No more Solo cups or pouring from whatever was cheapest. I knew the difference between Pinot Grigio and Sauvignon Blanc. I'd become that girl, the one who knew what to pair with pasta and which bottle to bring to a party.

One night, while Ashley and I were working on our capstone project, I poured myself another glass. She watched me, eyebrows raised.

"You drink more than most people I know," she said.

"It helps me think," I told her, without missing a beat. That line had become my go-to. "And besides, I'm not getting drunk. Just maintaining a pleasant buzz."

She gave me a look but didn't say anything else. Nobody ever really did. This was college, and college was supposed to be a little excessive. We were young. We were invincible. Hangovers were just part of the culture. Consequences were something we'd think about later.

By the time I hit graduation, I could drink most of the guys under the table and still make it to class the next morning. I knew how to plan it out. When to stop, when to switch to water, when to chew gum or pop a mint. I'd even figured out that vodka left less of a smell than beer, which came in handy when I needed to be discreet.

I thought of it as a skill. Something I'd mastered.

The morning of graduation, I woke up on Jake's couch with a skull-cracking headache and flashes of the night before playing in fragments. There was champagne at the honors reception. Then a rooftop party. Then Murphy's Pub. At some point, shots. At some point, dancing. At some point, forgetting.

Jake walked in holding a mug of coffee and a couple of aspirins.

"How are you feeling?" he asked, smirking like he already knew.

"Like I partied my way through the best four years of my life," I said, smiling despite the headache.

Later that day, dressed in my cap and gown, I stood among a sea of bright futures while the dean gave a speech about ambition and dreams and making a difference. I felt proud. Hopeful. I got a degree. A boyfriend. Job prospects. I'd made it through.

More than that, I'd figured out how to navigate life. I could handle pressure. I could hold a conversation with anyone. I could push through loneliness, boredom, anxiety, and stress. I had a secret weapon. A glass of wine could turn any night into something worth remembering, or at least something I didn't mind forgetting.

As the caps flew into the air and the cheering started, I didn't realize what I was walking away with. Not just a diploma in communications, but something else I hadn't planned on picking up.

I was graduating with a minor in functional alcoholism.

But I didn't see it like that then.

All I knew was, whatever came next, I had wine to help me handle it.

Chapter Three

Love, Marriage, and Wine Glasses

JAKE AND I POPPED a bottle of champagne the night we moved into our first apartment together. The place was still full of cardboard boxes, but we were giddy with the kind of optimism that made even an unfinished space feel like home.

"To us," he said, raising his glass.

"To our first place," I replied, clinking mine against his.

Looking back now, I'm not sure which of us had less of a clue what we were actually celebrating.

The apartment was a third-floor walkup in a building full of other fresh-out-of-college couples trying to look more grown-up than they felt. It had creaky hardwood floors, windows that let in too much cold air, and a kitchen that could fit two people if one of them didn't mind being pinned to the fridge.

We didn't mind. We liked being that close.

The early days felt like the opening credits of a romantic comedy. Jake would come home from his entry-level job at the investment firm, loosen his tie, and tell me stories from the office. I'd talk about my marketing coordinator job and whatever new coworker drama had unfolded that day. Sometimes I cooked. Sometimes we ordered Thai or pizza. Either way, we lit candles because we didn't have proper lamps yet, and it made even cheap dinners feel like something more.

Wine just sort of happened. It started with a glass here and there, paired with pasta or pad Thai, a little something to unwind. One night I said, "We should get a wine rack."

Jake looked around at our sad little kitchen, then back at me. "Very adult of us," he said.

"We are adults," I reminded him, even though I still felt like I was playing house.

"Then we definitely need a wine rack."

By the end of the week, we had one. Just a small wooden thing that held six bottles, but I treated it like it belonged in a magazine spread. I started reading wine blogs. Learned the difference between dry and fruity. Learned which bottle to open with salmon, which with stir-fry. Jake handled the budgeting. I handled the wine. It felt like a fair deal.

A glass with dinner became part of our rhythm. A reward at the end of a long workday. A little ritual that made everything feel more like what I thought adulthood should look like. We'd sit at our tiny table, sip slowly, and talk about our five-year plan like we had any idea where we were going.

"I love this," Jake said one night, reaching for my hand. We were halfway through our second bottle, toasting his first work bonus.

"The wine?" I asked, smiling.

"This. Us. All of it."

Wine made it easier to believe we'd stay like that forever.

By the time our one-year lease was up, wine had become as much a part of our evenings as checking the mail or flipping through Netflix. I'd start drinking while cooking. One glass while chopping vegetables. Another while waiting for the oven timer. By the time Jake walked in the door, I already felt the day melting away.

"How was your day?" was a question best answered with wine in hand.

Then one evening, Jake watched me refill my third glass and said, casually, "You might want to slow down a little."

It landed harder than he probably intended. My cheeks flushed before I could respond. "What's that supposed to mean?"

He softened right away. "Nothing bad. I've just noticed we've both been drinking more lately. I just don't want us to fall into bad habits, that's all."

"Bad habits?" My voice went high without warning. "We're having wine with dinner. That's what couples do. That's normal."

"I know," he said, reaching for my hand.

I pulled it away.

"Forget it," he added quickly. "I'm probably overthinking it."

I tried to forget it, but I couldn't. That night, every sip felt observed. Every time I lifted my glass, I wondered if he was counting. I started listening to changes in his voice, scanning his expression for judgment. Even when he said nothing, I felt it.

The argument that followed wasn't really about wine. It was about trust, freedom, and the feeling of being watched in my own home. I told him he didn't understand how stressful work had become. I accused him of trying to turn me into someone I wasn't.

He apologized. Said he loved me just the way I was. Said he'd never bring it up again.

And he didn't. For a while.

But something shifted after that. A small crack in what had felt like solid ground. I became more aware of my drinking... not in the sense of stopping, but in the sense of timing it better. I poured my first glass before he got home. Sipped slower at dinner. Waited until he was in the shower or zoned out in front of the TV before pouring the next one.

I told myself it wasn't hiding. It was being considerate. Why make him worry about something that wasn't a problem?

I had it under control. I was functioning. I was managing stress. I was still the woman he loved.

And I wasn't ready to admit I'd already crossed a line I couldn't see.

Two years into living together, Jake proposed.

He picked a romantic Italian restaurant where we'd had our first real date. I knew something was up. He'd been jittery all week and made the reservation with a formality that didn't match our usual routine. Still, I hadn't expected it to happen quite like that.

I hadn't expected to be a little drunk.

I'd poured myself a glass of wine before we even left the apartment. Work had been brutal that day, and I needed something to take the edge off. When we sat down at the restaurant, Jake ordered a bottle for the table. Something nicer than usual, the kind we saved for holidays or promotions.

"To us," he said, raising his glass, just like he always did.

"To us," I echoed. The champagne bubbles tickled my throat, and I giggled.

The whole evening was perfect. Warm light, smooth wine, and Jake looking at me like I was his whole world. The conversation flowed without effort, the way it always did with him when we were both a little buzzed. I felt light, happy, like the best version of myself.

By the time dessert came, I was relaxed enough to miss all the clues. I didn't see it coming until he pushed back his chair, got down on one knee, and pulled out a ring.

"Emily," he said, voice a little shaky, "will you marry me?"

The ring sparkled. His eyes were glassy. The moment felt like a dream.

"Yes," I blurted out, before he'd even finished.

The restaurant burst into applause. Someone at the next table shouted for champagne. A waiter brought more glasses, and suddenly we were surrounded by strangers cheering and raising their drinks in our honor. It felt like a movie scene. Too good to be real.

I couldn't tell you how much I drank that night. I just remember floating. Everything shimmered. Everything tasted sweet and felt golden. This was what love was supposed to feel like. This was what forever looked like.

Then came the bachelorette party.

We booked a weekend in Napa. Of course we did. A bride obsessed with wine celebrating her last days of singlehood in wine country practically wrote itself.

The plan was wine tastings, massages, laughter, and memories. What I didn't plan for was realizing I had no idea how to stop.

By the fourth winery, I was stumbling. It was barely past two in the afternoon.

"Maybe eat something," Ashley suggested gently, looping her arm through mine.

"I'm fine," I said, but my words were slipping into each other. "It's my bachelorette party. I'm supposed to get drunk."

"Drunk, yeah. But not passed out," Jennifer added. She was always the practical one.

I wasn't unconscious. I was very much awake. And everything felt hilarious. Everything felt beautiful. I felt beautiful. Loved. Free.

It was only later that things spiraled. I ended the night on the hotel bathroom floor, crying in the toilet, my dress bunched around my knees. Ashley held my hair back while I sobbed about how much I loved Jake, how lucky I was, how perfect everything would be.

"You're going to be such a good wife," she said, rubbing my back as my stomach finally calmed.

"I just want to be perfect for him," I whispered.

"You already are," she whispered back.

And at that moment, I believed her. Because the wine told me it was true.

The next morning, I woke up with the kind of hangover that makes you question your life choices. My head pounded, my mouth felt like sandpaper, and I had no idea how I'd gotten back to the hotel. None. It was like someone had cut an entire reel of film out of my brain.

Ashley filled in the blanks over breakfast while I sat there in oversized sunglasses, nursing a coffee I couldn't stomach. She laughed as she told me how I'd cried on the sidewalk about how much I loved Jake, how I'd begged her to let me call him at two in the morning.

"You told him you missed his face," she said, shaking her head like it was adorable. "Classic bride behavior. You're allowed to go a little crazy."

I forced a laugh, but my stomach twisted. I'd blacked out. Fully. Completely. There were entire hours I couldn't account for, and it scared the hell out of me. I'd never lost time like that before. The idea that there were moments (conversations, actions, memories) that belonged to me but weren't accessible unsettled me in a way I couldn't explain.

But then again, it was my bachelorette party. If there was ever a time to go too far, this was it. Right?

We celebrated a lot, those first few months after the marriage. Jake's promotion. My campaign launch. Our three-month anniversary. A random snowstorm. The Oscars. Tuesday night. We could turn anything into an occasion. Finding a reason to open a bottle was never hard.

The problems started when Jake's job shifted.

"It's just a few months," he said, pointing to the calendar he'd printed with his travel schedule. "Once we land with this client, everything will slow down."

Three nights a week, he was gone. Hotel rooms and redeye flights became part of his routine. And just like that, I was alone.

The first night he left, I ordered pizza and put on a rom-com, convincing myself I was fine. Independent. Sophisticated, even. I poured a glass of wine before dinner and another with it. I told myself it was no big deal.

The second night Jake was gone. I opened a bottle to go with leftover Chinese food. Eating alone felt too bleak without something to soften the edges.

By the end of that week, I had a routine. I'd come home from work, kick off my shoes, change into something soft and forgiving, open a bottle, and settle in with takeout and whatever show Jake usually rolled his eyes at. It felt indulgent in a way that passed for self-care. Like something a busy, grown-up woman was entitled to. Like something a wife, temporarily on her own, deserved.

"How are you handling your alone time?" Jake asked one night during his usual check-in.

"Fine," I said, and it was mostly true. "Just relaxing. Catching up on all the shows you hate."

There was a pause. Then... "Are you drinking by yourself?"

He didn't sound angry. It wasn't an accusation. But I heard something else in his voice, something I didn't want to name.

"Just a glass of wine with dinner," I told him.

That was also true, technically. I just didn't mention that "a glass" had turned into "a bottle." Or that "with dinner" now meant before dinner, during dinner, and long after I'd finished eating.

Wine disappeared faster when I was drinking alone. A bottle that used to last us two or three nights was gone in one. I found myself stopping at the wine shop more often, always with an excuse ready. Hosting friends. Stocking up for the weekend. Bringing a bottle to someone's house.

The woman at the counter started to recognize me. "Another party?" She asked one Thursday as I placed three bottles on the counter.

"Just restocking," I said with a practiced smile, like I was picking up eggs or paper towels.

And honestly, by then, it felt that routine.

The first time I hid a bottle, I told myself it was just for convenience.

Jake had been away on a three-day trip. My work week had been brutal. I'd finished the open bottle the night before and figured we'd want something to share when he got home. So, I bought two. One to replace the empty, and one extra. Just in case.

Except when he walked in and saw two new bottles, I panicked. If he did the math, it wouldn't add up. Not in a way I could explain.

So, I tucked one in the garage, behind a bin of tangled Christmas lights. The other went in the kitchen, opened and waiting by the time he kicked off his shoes.

"I missed this," Jake said that night, pulling me close on the couch with his wine glass in hand. "I missed us."

"I did too," I said, and I meant it. Being with Jake was better than drinking alone. But drinking alone was still better than being alone without anything at all.

That bottle in the garage sat untouched for three weeks. Then one night, after another awful day at work and another voicemail from my boss that made my stomach knot, I remembered it. I didn't feel like getting in the car or facing the store clerk again. I didn't need to.

I already had what I needed.

It felt like a small win, having a backup. Like I was prepared. Like I had some kind of control.

After that, I started keeping extras in other places too. Behind the winter coats in the hall closet, in the pantry behind a tower of paper towels, in the trunk of my car, just in case.

I told myself it wasn't hiding. I was just staying organized. Ready for anything.

"You've been drinking more lately," Jake said one night, watching me pour my third glass during dinner.

"Have I?" I kept my tone light, feeling surprised. Inside, my chest tightened.

"Maybe it's just me," he said, but he didn't look convinced. "I've been gone so much. Maybe I'm just more aware of it when I'm back."

"Maybe you should drink more," I said, trying to laugh. "Catch up with your wife."

He smiled, but it didn't reach his eyes. "Maybe I should."

But he didn't. Jake nursed his one beer or single glass of wine while I emptied mine and quietly reached for more. When he was around, I drank faster, tried to match his pace and pretended I was satisfied. When he wasn't paying attention, I'd top off my glass or sneak another. And when he left for his next trip, I poured freely again, slipping back into my routine like it had been waiting for me.

And in a way, it had.

I started finishing my first glass while cooking dinner, before Jake got home. That way, we could begin the evening together with fresh drinks, and he wouldn't notice I was already ahead.

Work happy hours became an extension of my evening routine, not a replacement. What used to be occasional turned into something I relied on. Tuesday wine with coworkers, Thursday cocktails with clients, Friday drinks to celebrate surviving the week.

"You're becoming quite the socialite," Jake said one morning when I mentioned my third happy hour of the week.

"It's networking," I told him. "Building relationships. It's good for my career."

That part was true. My boss had started to notice how easily I connected with clients, how I could take a stiff meeting and turn it into something relaxed, even fun. Over drinks, I was charming and confident. I knew how to listen, when to smile, how to make people feel seen.

What I didn't mention was how much I needed those drinks. How they took the edge off before I even got home. How showing up with a soft buzz made it easier to keep that perfect level of calm through the rest of the evening. If I started at happy hour, I didn't have to drink as much in front of Jake. The math worked in my favor.

Until the night he showed up.

"I thought I'd crash your party," Jake said, suddenly beside me at the bar. I was ordering my third martini.

"Jake!" I threw my arms around him, caught somewhere between surprise and panic. My voice came out too loud. I felt my balance tip as I leaned into him. "What are you doing here?"

"Missing my wife," he said. He smiled, but his eyes moved past me. Taking in the drinks lined up on the bar, the flushed faces, the way I leaned on the counter for support.

"Let me introduce you to everyone," I said quickly, grabbing his hand, trying to steer the moment, trying to pretend I was less drunk than I was.

The rest of the night blurred. Names I couldn't quite pronounce. Conversations I couldn't quite follow. Jake standing just behind me, silent but tense in that way I'd come to dread.

We didn't talk about it on the way home. We didn't talk about it before bed. But the next morning, over coffee, he broke the silence.

"Emily," he said gently, "I think we need to talk about your drinking."

I stared at the table. "What about it?"

"You were pretty drunk last night," he said. "At a work event."

"I was socializing," I told him. "That's what happy hour is for."

"Not like that," he said. "Not to that extent."

"What does that even mean?"

He ran his hands through his hair. "It means I'm worried. About how often you're drinking. About how it's starting to affect everything else. "

My mouth went dry. My stomach twisted with that mix of nausea and panic that always followed a heavy night.

I wanted to argue. To tell him he was overreacting. To remind him of the dinners and the toasts and the way wine had always been part of our life together. To insist I was fine.

Instead, I cried.

"I'm not an alcoholic," I said, the words tasting sharp and metallic. "I have a good job. I'm responsible. I'm a good wife."

"I know," Jake said quickly, reaching for my hand. "I'm not saying you are. I'm just saying maybe we should both slow down. Maybe take a break from drinking. Just for a while."

"A break?" The word landed like punishment.

"Just a few weeks," he said. "See how it feels."

I nodded. I said yes because I loved him. Because I needed to prove I could. Because admitting how scared I felt without it was worse than anything he could say.

To my surprise, I made it three weeks.

Three full weeks without a drop of alcohol. No wine with dinner, no champagne at celebrations, no beer at barbecues. I clenched my way through work stress with herbal tea and deep breathing. I went to two office happy hours and ordered club soda with lime, bracing myself for humiliation that never came. It didn't kill me.

By the end of week three, I felt triumphant. Strong. Like I'd proved something not just to Jake, but to myself.

"See?" I told him one evening while we cooked dinner together, both of us holding glasses of sparkling water. "I can stop anytime I want. It's really not that hard. I'm not an alcoholic."

"I'm proud of you," he said, and I could see relief soften his face. "How do you feel?"

"Great," I told him, and I meant it. "Clearer. More energetic. I don't even know why I thought I needed wine to relax."

That confidence was its own kind of intoxication. I felt untouchable, like I'd conquered alcohol. I could take it or leave it, and I had just spent three weeks proving it.

Which is exactly why I felt so comfortable reaching for "just one glass" at my college friend's birthday party the next weekend.

"You sure?" Jake asked when I picked up a flute of champagne from the waiter's tray.

"It's a special occasion," I said, raising the glass toward the birthday girl. "And I've already proven I can stop anytime I want. Three weeks, remember?"

The champagne slid down like victory. Like vindication. I told myself I was drinking like a normal person again socially, moderately, without need.

But normal people don't spend three weeks obsessing about not drinking. Normal people don't feel triumphant about ordering club soda. Normal people don't carry alcohol around in their thoughts even when their hands are empty.

Normal people also don't go from one toast of champagne to polishing off a full bottle of wine at home, convincing themselves they'd earned it after such impressive self-control.

That break hadn't cured me. It tricked me. It convinced me that willpower was enough, that I could manage my drinking by sheer discipline. And that false confidence was the most dangerous delusion of all.

Because now I believed I could stop anytime I wanted. Which also meant I believed I never had to stop for good.

One night, Jake and I sat on the back deck, a bottle of white between us. The sky was pink. The air smelled like fresh-cut grass and possibility.

"Are you happy?" he asked.

"So happy," I said. And I was. At least, I wanted to be.

We had everything we were supposed to want. The house. The careers. The love story people envied. The Facebook photos to prove it. Sunsets in Tuscany, date nights in Napa, dinner parties with perfect lighting and better wine.

"Perfect couple," the comments said. "Living the dream."

And we were. Sort of.

The problem was that the dream needed more and more wine to keep it from slipping through my fingers. I wasn't drinking to escape a nightmare. I was drinking to stay inside the fantasy.

The night Jake came home early from his latest trip, I wasn't ready. Not for him, not for the moment, not for the look I didn't see coming.

I'd spent the day cleaning, scrubbing baseboards, fluffing pillows, and lighting candles I usually ignored. I wanted the house to feel warm and welcoming. I wanted him to walk in and see effort, love, and pride.

But I'd also been drinking. Just a little at first, a glass while folding laundry. Then another with lunch. Then, just enough to keep the edges smooth, the rhythm steady. It made everything easier. Calmer. More pleasant.

By the time I heard his key in the door, I had several glasses in. Enough to feel light and loose. Enough that my heart jumped. Not just from excitement, but from panic.

"Surprise!" he called, his voice echoing down the hallway as his suitcase thudded against the floor. "My meeting got canceled. I caught an earlier flight."

I found him in the living room and wrapped my arms around him like it had been months. My voice was too bright. My smile was too big.

"I missed you so much," I said. That part was real.

"I can tell," he said.

I pulled back, a sudden chill running through me. His look wasn't mean, or even suspicious. It was quiet. Too quiet. Like he already knew. Like I didn't need to say anything because the truth was sitting between us.

"How was your flight?" I asked, trying to steer us somewhere safer.

"Fine." He didn't smile. He didn't accuse. He just looked at me, and the weight of it made my stomach turn. "How was your day?"

"Good. Productive. I got a lot done around the house."

His eyes swept over the freshly vacuumed carpet, the polished coffee table, the throw blanket folded like a store display. "Yeah. It looks great."

But his gaze didn't stay in the room. It came back to me. And in it, I saw something new.

Not anger. Not disappointment.

Tired. Like maybe he'd stopped hoping anything would change.

That night, I lay next to him in bed, staring at the ceiling, listening to his steady breathing. It was even and calm, like he was already somewhere far from me. Somewhere I couldn't reach.

And all I could think about was that look. The way he saw straight through me. The way I'd become someone he didn't recognize.

So, I made myself a promise.

I will change and be different. I'd get it together. I'd prove to him and to myself that I was still the woman he married. The one who used to make him laugh, who lit up when he walked in the room. The one who didn't need a glass in her hand to belong in her own life.

I'd show him our life was still good. Still worth it. Still, something we could save.

But before I had the chance to prove anything (before I could even try), life threw something at me I never saw coming.

Chapter Four

Two Under Two and a Bottle Under the Sink

I HADN'T EVEN FINISHED peeing on the stick when the two pink lines appeared.

Bold. Immediate. No room for doubt.

Pregnant.

I stared at the test, my hands trembling, heart pounding so hard it drowned out everything else. After two years of marriage and a hundred late-night "someday" conversations, it was finally real. We were going to have a baby.

My first reaction was joy. The kind that catches in your throat. I could already see little feet pattering down the hallway, a nursery filled with soft blankets and impossibly tiny clothes.

But right behind the joy came something else. Something colder.

Terror.

Not the kind that comes with big life changes. Not bottles, diapers, or sleepless nights. I was terrified of something far more immediate.

I was terrified to stop drinking.

"Jake!" I called from the bathroom floor, the test still in my hand like it might vanish if I blinked. "Can you come here?"

He appeared in the doorway like he'd been waiting for this moment forever. His eyes went straight to the test, then to me, and he lit up.

"Really?" he asked, even though the answer was written in bold pink right there.

"Really," I said.

He lifted me off the floor and spun me around in our cramped bathroom, both of us laughing like kids, high on joy and disbelief.

"We're going to be parents," he whispered, kissing my forehead.

"We're going to be parents," I echoed, and suddenly the words felt massive. Beautiful. Terrifying.

That night, Jake opened a nice bottle of champagne. One we'd been saving. He poured two glasses, and I just... stared at mine.

It sat on the counter like it had turned to poison.

"I guess I can't have this anymore," I said, trying to sound breezy.

"Not for nine months," Jake smiled, raising his glass. "To our baby, and to my amazing wife who's giving up wine for a year."

I lifted my glass of sparkling cider. "To our baby," I said, forcing a smile as I took a sip that tasted like regret.

Nine months. I could do that. Millions of women did it. Just a season. Just until the baby came.

How hard could it be?

Harder than I ever imagined.

The first month, I got a free pass. Morning sickness hit like a truck. I couldn't keep anything down. Not even the thought of wine. The smell alone made me gag. I lived on ginger ale and saltines, curled up on the couch in sweatpants, too sick to care.

"Silver lining," I told Jake one night, picking at a piece of dry toast. "At least I'm too nauseated to miss drinking."

"Nature's detox plan," he joked, rubbing my back while I tried not to throw up.

But by the second month, the sickness eased. And what took its place wasn't relief. It was anxiety. Low-level, constant, never shutting off. About the baby. About money. About whether we were ready. About everything.

And I knew exactly what could quiet it.

Unlike the last time I quit alcohol for three weeks on sheer willpower, this was different. The pressure of pregnancy, the fear about the baby, the endless knot of stress and uncertainty... all of it made the temptation stronger than ever. My willpower wasn't enough this time.

Just one glass.

One glass to smooth the edges. One glass to slow the noise in my head.

"Pregnant women in Europe drink wine," I whispered to myself one night while Jake worked late. "They say it helps digestion."

I pulled out a bottle of red I'd been saving for a special occasion. Poured a splash. Just a taste.

The first sip felt like a warm hug. Like finally exhaling after holding my breath for weeks.

One sip became two. Then three. Then the glass was empty, and I poured another.

I wasn't drunk. I wasn't even tipsy. I was just... okay.

And then came the guilt.

I spent the rest of the night glued to my phone, scrolling medical sites, desperate to find proof that one glass wasn't a big deal. That the baby would be fine. That I wasn't already failing at motherhood.

The internet wasn't reassuring.

I dumped the rest of the bottle down the sink and watched it swirl away like a secret.

Never again, I told myself.

Three days later, it happened again. Then again, next week.

Each time, I made a promise. Each time, I broke it. Each time, I convinced myself it wasn't enough to cause harm. And each time, I told myself this was the last time.

I wasn't drinking to get drunk. I wasn't drinking every day. I was drinking when I was scared, overwhelmed, or losing my grip on the person I was supposed to be.

And even then, I knew that was a problem I couldn't explain away.

Emma Grace Matthews was born on a crisp October morning, after fourteen hours of labor I somehow survived completely sober.

She came out slippery and screaming and heartbreakingly perfect. When the doctor laid her on my chest, something in me cracked open. It wasn't just love. It was something fiercer. My body knew nothing would ever matter more than this tiny girl in my arms.

Jake's face crumpled with joy. "She's beautiful," he whispered, tears sliding down his cheeks. "You did amazing, sweetheart. Look what you did."

I looked down at her, at our daughter, and everything else faded away. I wasn't tired. I wasn't scared. The world around us disappeared.

And in that sacred, breathless moment, I made a promise.

I would be the mother she deserved.

I would protect her from the world, from danger, from anything that had ever hurt me.

And especially from me. From my own worst habits. From the part of me I had never fully controlled.

I would stop drinking. For real this time. Forever, if that's what it took.

That promise lasted six weeks.

Those first weeks were beautiful, yes but also brutal. A blur of 3 a.m. feedings, endless diaper changes, and the kind of bone-deep exhaustion that feels like you're losing pieces of your mind.

Jake took paternity leave, thank God, because I couldn't have done it alone. Even with both of us, some days felt like we were barely staying afloat.

One morning after Emma cried for three straight hours despite being fed, changed, rocked, sung to, swaddled, and walked in desperate loops around the apartment, I collapsed on the couch, clutching a cold cup of coffee like a life raft.

"How are people supposed to do this?" I asked Jake, my voice cracking.

"I have no idea," he admitted, eyes hollow.

"Maybe we're doing it wrong," I said. **"Maybe we're not cut out for this."**

He looked at me seriously. "We are. We just have to make it through the change."

The "change," it turned out, made sobriety feel less like a noble promise and more like a cruel joke.

I couldn't relax. Every time Emma cried, my chest went into full-blown panic. Every feeding felt like a test I hadn't studied for. Even when she slept, I lay awake staring at the monitor, convinced I'd miss the moment she stopped breathing. I read SIDS articles until my brain spun. Googled "how to know if baby is getting enough milk" thirty times a day. Second-guessed everything from swaddle tightness to whether my singing voice was soothing enough.

I had never needed a drink more in my life. And I had never been more unable to have one.

"You should have a glass of wine," my mom said one day during a visit. "It'll help you relax. A relaxed mom makes better milk."

"Mom, I'm breastfeeding," I reminded her, already frayed.

"One glass won't hurt. In my day, the doctor recommended wine. Said it helped with let-down."

I knew better. At least, I thought I did. But her words stuck like a splinter.

Because I was desperate. Desperate for something, anything, that would help me feel normal again. Not blissful mom-normal. Just human. Just steady enough to keep going without crying in the laundry room every night.

That night, after Emma finally went down and Jake buried himself in a project, I stood in the kitchen staring at the wine rack like it had something to say.

I didn't pour much. Just a small glass. Barely two fingers. Enough to take the edge off, to soften the sharpness of the day.

My shoulders had been up near my ears for weeks, my chest tight like I hadn't taken a real breath since labor. That first sip was instant relief. Like my nervous system exhaled for the first time in months.

I felt... okay. Capable. Calmer. Like maybe I could manage this whole motherhood thing after all.

Then, two hours later, Emma woke up.

She was hungry, fussing softly in the dark, her warm little body curling into mine as I settled into the rocking chair. I watched her nurse, her tiny mouth latched to me, and I knew...knew that there was alcohol in my milk. Not much. Just a trace. But it was there, and the thought sat like a stone in my gut.

She seemed fine. Sleepy. Peaceful. Perfect. But I couldn't un-know what I knew.

The next morning, I pumped and dumped. Poured an entire bag of milk down the sink, pretending it was about responsibility, not about covering my tracks. Telling myself I was doing both, protecting her and protecting my sanity. I needed to be okay too, right? Wasn't that part of being a good mom?

It felt like a reasonable compromise.

By the time Emma was three months old, I had a system. Feed her before bedtime. Have my glass of wine. Dump the first milk in the morning. Repeat.

It was predictable. Manageable. And it made me feel like I hadn't completely lost myself to burp cloths and bottle warmers.

Jake noticed, of course. He didn't say much. Just gave me that quiet, unreadable look when I poured my nightly glass.

"Everything okay?" he'd ask lightly.

"Just trying to relax a little," I'd say. "Parenting's no joke."

"You're doing great," he'd tell me. And I think he meant it. But more than once, I caught him scrolling on his phone, searching things like "breastfeeding and alcohol" or "postpartum anxiety", and pretending he wasn't.

When Emma was eight months old, I saw that second pink line again.

This time, there was no joy. No tears. No laughter. Just me, sitting there holding the pregnancy test like it was a verdict.

Pregnant. Again.

Emma wasn't even one yet. I was still figuring out how to be a mother to one baby. How to stay sane, stay married, stay afloat and now there would be two. Two babies under two. Two nap schedules. Two highchairs. Two car seats. Two years, minimum, of no drinking.

I tried to smile when I handed Jake the test.

"Surprise," I said, my voice was all wrong.

His eyes widened. "Already?" Then came the flickers. Surprise, joy, panic, something like fear. "Wow. That's... wow."

"Irish twins," I mumbled, trying to make it sound like a joke instead of a slow-motion scream.

"That's wonderful," Jake said, but his voice cracked just enough for me to hear the doubt under it.

This pregnancy hit harder than the first. My body didn't get a break. I was already exhausted, chasing a crawling baby, barely sleeping, still breastfeeding. There was no glowing second trimester. Just nausea, back pain, and stress stacked on stress.

And this time, I didn't have the same resolve.

The first drink came after a hellish day. Emma teething, screaming like she was in pain, me nauseated and lightheaded, barely holding it together. Jake texted he'd be late. Again.

I looked at the wine fridge and told myself. Just one glass. Just enough to keep from breaking tonight.

The guilt hit before I finished it.

I knew better. I'd read every article, every cautionary blog, every terrifying paragraph about fetal alcohol spectrum disorder. I knew the risk was low but still real and that I was doing it anyway.

But in that moment, spiraling into a full-on breakdown felt just as dangerous. What good was I to Emma, to this baby, to Jake, if I cracked under the pressure?

I told myself it was a calculated choice. That one glass here and there was the lesser of two evils.

That it didn't make me a bad mother.

That it made me functional.

And in a strange, messed-up way... that felt like enough.

By my second trimester, "occasional" had quietly become "regular."

One glass every few days turned into one most nights. And on the hard days when Emma refused to nap or Lucas twisted like a corkscrew in my belly. Sometimes two. I needed something to take the edge off the chaos, something to make me feel like I was still a person and not just a machine that breastfed, wiped noses, and kept everyone alive.

I told myself it was fine. I scoured the internet for anything to back me up. Studies on French women, blogs about "relaxed pregnancies," forums full of moms swearing a little wine never hurt their kids. I absorbed it like gospel. Clung to the idea that stress might be worse than a few sips of wine. That this was, in its own way, self-care.

I became an expert in justifying what I already wanted to do.

Then Lucas James Matthews arrived, red-faced and wailing, in the middle of a February snowstorm. Fourteen hours of labor and there he was. Tiny, healthy, perfect. I held him to my chest, skin to skin, just like I had with Emma, and the same rush of blinding love poured through me.

But this time, under the awe and joy, there was something else.

Relief.

Relief that he looked okay. That nothing seemed wrong. That maybe, just maybe, I'd gotten away with it.

"Two under two," Jake said, cradling Lucas like glass while Emma ran wild around the hospital room. His voice was soft with wonder, but I could hear the panic.

"We can do this," I said, trying to sound like I believed it.

"We can definitely do this," he echoed, but he looked like he was convincing himself too.

What came next wasn't just hard. It was soul-splitting.

Emma was still very much a baby. She needed constant eyes on her so she wouldn't climb or drop something on Lucas. She needed attention and reassurance that she still mattered. Lucas needed to be fed every two hours. He had his days and nights reversed and cried like it was his job.

And me? I needed to heal from birth while running on three hours of sleep, pretending I had it together while wondering, every hour, if I was about to shatter.

The wine crept back in during Lucas's afternoon naps.

"Mommy needs a little break," I'd murmur to Emma, settling her with blocks or a muted cartoon. Then I'd pour a glass and sit quietly, staring at nothing while she babbled nearby. That glass gave me thirty minutes of quiet in my head. It softened the panic. It gave me the illusion I was managing.

It became the only part of the day that felt bearable.

Then Jake found the sippy cup.

I was upstairs bathing the kids, trying to keep soap out of Emma's eyes and Lucas from screaming, when he called from the kitchen.

"Emily?"

His voice had that tone. Half curious, half serious. I froze.

"Yeah?"

"Why does Emma's sippy cup smell like wine?"

Time stopped. My body went cold.

"What?" I said, too quickly.

"This pink one," he said, holding it up. "It smells like wine."

I stared at the tub, my heart pounding. I remembered. That day, I'd poured a glass half-asleep and grabbed the wrong cup. I'd caught it before handing it to her, rinsed it fast, and told myself no harm done.

Now here it was. Proof.

"I probably used it while cooking," I said flatly. "Like to measure something. And forgot to wash it."

He looked at the cup. Looked at me. Said nothing for a long moment. Then nodded and ran it under hot water again. Carefully. Thoroughly.

He didn't push. But I saw something shift in him.

He was starting to wonder what else I wasn't telling him.

And honestly? So was I.

The bedtime stories started slurring together sometime around the fourth month.

It wasn't intentional. I didn't set out to drink while putting the kids to bed. But that evening glass of wine kept creeping earlier. First after bedtime. Then after dinner. Then with dinner. Before long, I was sipping while flipping pancakes, sipping while warming bottles, sipping while reading about sleepy bunnies and magical trains.

"Once upon a time," I'd start, Emma tucked under one arm, Lucas dozing on my shoulder, "there was a little princess who lived in a... in a..."

The words blurred. My tongue felt slow. My brain lagged behind the sentences. Emma didn't notice. She was too focused on the pictures, but I noticed. I was reading bedtime stories to my babies with wine on my breath.

And this was exactly the kind of thing I'd sworn I would never, ever do.

I noticed. And I kept doing it anyway.

The mornings were the worst. Lucas would start squirming and grunting at five-thirty, ready to nurse. I'd peel myself off the pillow, head pounding, mouth dry, stomach turning. Emma would appear in the kitchen an hour later, rubbing her eyes and asking for pancakes. Or eggs. Or anything that required more energy than I had.

"Mommy sick?" she asked once, clutching her favorite stuffed animal.

"No, baby," I told her. "Just tired." I set a bowl of cereal in front of her and tried to smile.

But it wasn't just "tired". It was hungover. It was shame. It was the weight of being the only caretaker for two babies while quietly unraveling.

Jake started working longer hours around then. He said things at the firm were "busy," but I knew better. I think he couldn't stand coming home to the mess. To me. To the wine glasses in the sink and the barely contained mayhem of our life.

I didn't blame him. I wanted to escape too. I just had a different method.

The afternoon everything cracked open was a Wednesday in September. One of those days that starts sideways and just keeps going. Emma was eighteen months old, furious because I'd given her the yellow cup instead of the purple one. Lucas was screaming, flailing, refusing to latch. And I was holding both of them while sobbing into a burp cloth, telling myself this wasn't how it was supposed to be.

So, I poured a glass of wine at two in the afternoon. I told myself it was medicinal. Just enough to calm down. Just enough to parent.

Ten minutes later, I was on the floor with Lucas in my arms and Emma stacking blocks beside me when it hit me. I felt... off. Not drunk, but not sober. Fuzzy. Like there was a thick pane of glass between me and the world.

And suddenly, I wasn't sure I could keep them safe.

What if I dropped Lucas? What if Emma slipped out the door? What if something happened and I couldn't react in time?

I called my mother.

"Can you come over?" I asked, trying to keep my voice steady. "I think I might be coming down with something. I don't want to get the kids sick."

She was there within twenty minutes. Took one look at me and gently scooped Lucas from my arms.

"You look awful," she said. "Go take a shower. I've got them."

I stood under the hot water and cried until my legs gave out.

I told myself I was a terrible mother. That I was failing the most important job I'd ever had. That I was choosing wine over safety, over clarity, over my kids.

And I decided I had to stop. For real this time. Not "cut back." Not "be more careful." Not "try to control it."

I had to stop.

That night, after the kids were asleep and the house was finally quiet, I sat at the kitchen table and wrote down every reason I needed to quit drinking.

Emma and Lucas deserved a mom who was present. Jake deserved a partner he could trust. I deserved to wake up without shame. I wanted to remember their childhoods. I wanted to be proud of myself. I wanted peace.

Two pages of reasons. Front and back.

Then I walked to our beautiful stainless steel wine fridge, the one I'd once designed the kitchen around. I pulled out every single bottle.

I poured them down the sink. Every single bottle.

Jake came home to find me barefoot in a sea of glass and red wine, the kitchen reeking of alcohol and resolve.

"What happened?" he asked, surveying the damage.

"I'm done," I said, my voice breaking. "I can't keep doing this."

He didn't ask questions. He didn't remind me I'd said that before. He just wrapped his arms around me and held on.

"We'll figure it out," he whispered. "Whatever you need, we'll figure it out."

And for the first time in months, I believed him.

I tried to quit so many times, but failed. This time, I believed I could quit. I believed love and willpower and motherhood would be enough. I believed I'd finally hit the turning point.

That night, I felt hope. Real hope.

Maybe I could do this. Maybe it wasn't too late. Maybe I could finally become the mother I promised I would be.

I just had to figure out how to live without the one thing I'd relied on for years.

How hard could it be?

Chapter Five

The Man Who Understood

COMING BACK TO WORK after maternity leave felt like returning to a city I used to live in. Familiar, but different in all the ways that mattered. I stood in the lobby that gray March morning, wrapped in a blazer that didn't quite fit, holding a breast pump bag that might as well have been a neon sign: New Mother Incoming.

Emma was 3 years old. Lucas, close to one. I'd had maybe three hours of sleep. And I was 10 months sober, still holding onto the promise I'd made the night I poured every bottle of wine down the sink with Jake standing beside me, no questions asked.

Some days, that promise felt like a gold medal. Other days, it felt like a straightjacket. That morning, it was both.

"Emily Matthews!"

Jessica from HR bounded over, all cheerful and corporate, the kind of smile people save for wedding receptions and first-day-back greetings. "Look at you! How does it feel to be back?"

"Surreal," I said. And it was surreal to pretend I was still the version of me who knew what she was doing.

She leaned in like she had a secret. "We've got someone new in marketing I think you'll click with. David Blake. Started while you were out. Great energy."

I nodded, barely listening. I just wanted to make it through the day without crying in a bathroom stall.

The break room used to be my little haven. Cheap coffee, quiet gossip, ten minutes to breathe. But that morning, it felt foreign. I stood in front of the coffee machine, staring at the buttons like they were in another language, wondering if I'd ever feel normal again.

"First day back?"

I turned. A man about my age stood behind me. Tall, sharp suit, kind face, dark hair, easy eyes. He looked at me not like I was broken, but like I was... human.

"That obvious?"

"The deer-in-headlights look gave it away," he said, smiling as he held out his hand. "David Blake. Started here about six months ago."

"Emily Matthews," I said, shaking it. He didn't ask if I was breastfeeding or how many ounces my baby was drinking. Refreshing.

"Need help with this thing?" He nodded toward the coffee machine. "It's moody. Worse-than-a-toddler moody."

"Please," I laughed, grateful for a normal adult exchange.

While he fiddled with the buttons, he glanced over. "How's it going? The return, I mean."

"It's... an adjustment," I said. "Feels like I'm trying to remember who I used to be."

He nodded, his expression softening. "I get that. I went through a divorce recently. You forget yourself, and then you start piecing things back together. It's disorienting, but freeing too."

That stopped me. He wasn't offering surface sympathy. He understood not the sleepless nights or leaking breasts, but the deeper unraveling. The grief of losing who you thought you were supposed to be.

"That must've been hard," I said.

"It was. Still is, sometimes. But you start asking different questions. Who do I want to be now? Not who I used to be. Not who I thought I should be. Just... now."

The coffee machine beeped. He handed me a steaming cup, and it felt like more than caffeine. It felt like permission.

"Thanks," I said. "For the coffee. And... the realness."

"Anytime," he smiled. "Give it a few weeks. You'll find your rhythm again."

I walked back to my desk holding more than coffee. For the first time in months, someone had seen me, not the mom version, not the barely-holding-it-together version. Just me. And instead of advice or pity, he'd given me something I hadn't realized I was starving for: understanding.

It didn't fix anything overnight. The next few weeks were still brutal, catching up on projects, relearning acronyms, surviving 4 PM Zoom meetings when all I wanted was to be home in sweatpants with my babies.

But it was lighter now. Less lonely.

David didn't save me. I wasn't looking to be saved. But in a sea of well-meaning people who only saw the chaos of my motherhood, he saw the woman inside it. And some days, that was enough.

He'd pop into my office with coffee when I looked ready to unravel. He caught me up on office gossip... who'd been promoted, who was secretly dating whom, who was about to quit. He told jokes that had nothing to do with teething or sleep regressions, and for the first time in months, I remembered what it felt like to laugh because something was actually funny.

More than anything, David never made me feel guilty for struggling.

"You know what you need?" he said one Thursday, stepping into my office while I sat surrounded by printouts and half-written notes, blinking back tears.

"A lobotomy?" I offered.

"A drink," he said with a grin.

The word hit like a slap.

I froze. "It's three o'clock."

"I meant after work," he chuckled, hands up. "There's a place around the corner. Low lights, real glasses, no toddlers throwing Cheerios. Just... peace. You look like you could use some peace."

I did. God, I did.

But the suggestion landed hard. Ten months sober. The longest I'd gone without alcohol since I was old enough to buy it. I'd made a promise to Jake, to the kids, to myself. I'd poured every bottle in our house down the sink like it was a ritual. I hadn't touched a drop since.

Still, standing there, looking at David's easy smile, his kind eyes, the way he saw me as someone who deserved peace... I felt the craving rise like a wave. Not just for the drink, but for the woman I used to be when I had one. Calm, collected, in control.

"I don't really drink anymore," I said finally. The words felt foreign, like they belonged to someone else.

"Really?" he said, blinking. But he didn't flinch or press. "They have good coffee."

I smiled.

"Or maybe," he added gently, "it's not about what you drink. Maybe it's just about stepping outside the pressure cooker for an hour. You don't have to earn rest, Emily. Especially not from your own life."

"I should probably go home," I said out of reflex. "The kids..."

"The kids will still be there in an hour," he said, soft but certain. "And they'll be better off with a mom who had sixty minutes to breathe."

He wasn't wrong. I was tired. Burned out. Trying to be perfect at everything (work, motherhood, marriage) and failing at all of it. Maybe I could go. Just for an hour. Just coffee. Just a break.

"Okay," I said. "One hour."

David smiled. "Just to unwind."

I told myself it was harmless. Just a small detour. Just a moment of escape.

But I knew, even then it was more than that.

It was a test. And I wasn't sure I'd pass.

Cellar Door was the kind of wine bar I used to love. Back when I was the version of myself who wore heels without resentment and chose wine by region instead of price. Exposed brick, candlelight, leather-bound menus. The kind of place that whispered, You're still young. You're still desirable. You still know who you are.

David led me to a table tucked into the far corner, well out of earshot from the after-work crowd. He looked comfortable here, like he'd been here enough times to know the best seat in the house.

The waitress came over, smiling, pad in hand. "What can I get you?"

My pulse spiked. My mouth opened.

"Just coffee," I said quickly. "Regular coffee."

David glanced at me, eyebrows raised, but didn't say anything. "Make that two," he told the waitress, handing her the menus.

I should have felt proud. Ten months sober, sitting in a wine bar and saying no.

Instead, it felt like being handed a participation trophy for a game I didn't want to play anymore.

"So," David said, settling into his seat, "what's making work feel like an uphill climb lately?"

I tried to focus on the conversation. We talked about deadlines, product launches, and how the internal approval process had turned into a Kafka novel. But while David spoke, my eyes drifted across the room.

At the next table, a woman laughed with her head tilted back, a glass of red wine in her hand, glowing like she'd just come back from vacation. She looked calm. Effortless. Like she hadn't wiped spit-up off her blouse that morning or googled "how to sleep-train two babies at once" during her lunch break.

I wanted to feel like that woman again. Just for an hour.

"You know what?" I said suddenly, cutting David off mid-sentence. "Actually... maybe I will have a glass of wine. Just one. It's been a long day."

He paused, something unreadable passing over his face. "Are you sure? You seemed pretty firm on the coffee."

"I was," I said. Then, without meaning to, added, "But I'm an adult. I can have a glass of wine after work. That's what normal adults do."

David raised a hand for the waitress. Didn't challenge me. Just waited.

"What do you recommend?" I asked when she arrived. My voice felt a little too loud, a little too bright.

"The Pinot Grigio's light and crisp," she said. "Nice way to unwind."

"Perfect," I replied, already ashamed of how relieved I sounded.

When the glass landed in front of me, I hesitated for a second, then took a sip.

The taste was instant nostalgia. Smooth, cool, familiar. Like slipping into an old pair of jeans that still fit. My shoulders loosened. My mind, always buzzing, quieted. I could breathe again.

David watched me. "Better?"

I smiled. "So much better. I'd forgotten what it felt like to relax."

But as the second sip went down, so did the guilt. It curled in. Slow and tight. I'd broken the streak. Broken the promise. Ten months gone. Just like that. Jake would be crushed if he knew. And the kids. God, the kids. Weren't they the reason I'd quit in the first place?

"Don't," David said gently.

"Don't what?"

"Don't turn this into a self-flagellation exercise. I can see it on your face. It's just a glass of wine. You're allowed to take care of yourself too."

That validation? It felt almost as good as the wine.

"My husband would disagree," I said, swirling the glass, trying not to sound bitter.

"He's not the one juggling two babies and a job and trying to reassemble her entire identity," David said, his voice low. "Where is he, anyway? Working late again?"

When I nodded, he continued, "Sometimes other people's rules don't apply when you're surviving. Especially when those other people aren't around to help."

The comment felt dangerous. Like a thought I'd had once but never dared say out loud.

We talked for two hours. About everything and nothing. Career detours, growing pains. He told me about his divorce in terms of how they'd wanted different lives and didn't realize it until they were already deep in one. I told him how motherhood had swallowed me whole. How I couldn't tell if I was grieving who I used to be or just exhausted.

He didn't flinch. He didn't offer platitudes. He listened. And when he looked at me, I didn't feel like a mess. I felt seen.

Not as a mother. Not as a wife. As a woman.

It had been so long since anyone looked at me that way. Like I was still in there somewhere. Still smart. Still interesting. Still desirable.

By my second glass of wine, I'd gotten too honest.

"I think Jake's checked out," I said. "He's been working late, avoiding the house. I don't blame him. I'm barely tolerable most days."

David leaned in slightly, close enough that I caught a whiff of cologne. Clean, subtle, expensive.

"Maybe he's giving you space to figure things out," he said.

"Or maybe he's realizing he married the wrong person."

David reached across the table and let his hand rest lightly on mine.

The touch was brief, but it lit up nerves I hadn't felt in years. Not romantic exactly, but intimate. Human. Like I was more than just the person who did the night feeds and managed everyone else's schedules.

"Emily," he said, his eyes intense, "anyone who's spent five minutes with you knows you're built for more than survival. You're special. Your husband should see that. You just need someone who recognizes your worth to help you find your balance again."

I didn't answer. Because I didn't know if he was right. But I wanted him to be.

It was the first time in months someone had seen more than what I'd become. David hadn't asked about sleep schedules or feeding routines. He hadn't glanced at his phone or offered parenting advice. He saw a woman. Tired, maybe, but still a woman with thoughts worth listening to and stories worth hearing.

When he said, "You're built for more than survival," I believed him.

I finished my wine and felt something I hadn't felt in a long time: like myself. Not the version of me who counted ounces of milk and measured her worth in nap schedules and patience. The other one. The woman who used to laugh easily, who had ambition and charm and confidence. The one who used to belong in places like Cellar Door.

"We should do this again," David said as we got up to leave.

"Definitely," I said. And I meant it.

Taking a taxi home, I felt a cocktail of emotions. One part euphoria, one part guilt, and a steady undercurrent of hunger. I wanted more. More of David's attention. More of that feeling. More of the easy, effortless version of myself I'd briefly been allowed to access.

Jake was on the couch with both babies when I walked in. Emma stacking blocks on the rug, Lucas asleep against his chest.

He looked exhausted, but peaceful. Steady in a way I hadn't been for a long time.

"How was work?" he asked, glancing up as I kicked off my heels.

"Good. Better than expected. I had to stay late with a colleague afterward. David Blake. He's new in marketing."

It wasn't a lie. Not exactly. But it wasn't the full story either. I left out drinking wine. I left out the way David's words had lingered with me. I left out how easily I'd broken the promise I'd made to myself, to Jake, to our children.

Jake smiled genuinely, I think. "That's great. You needed that."

I leaned down and kissed him. I picked up Emma and held her close, breathing in that familiar baby smell that always made my chest ache. Love mixed with responsibility, the way it always did. But tonight, there was something else too: a flicker of memory. The way David had looked at me across the table, curious and amused. The way I'd looked back.

"How were they?" I asked.

"Perfect angels," Jake said. "Emma ate her dinner. Lucas only fussed for twenty minutes. I even got some laundry done."

He said it like it was no big deal. Like keeping two babies alive and calm was just something you did. No drama. No collapse. He made it sound easy. And maybe for him, it was.

"You're natural at this," I said, settling Emma on my lap.

"So are you," he replied.

But his voice carried hesitation. As if he knew it wasn't quite true and was hoping if he said it out loud, it might become real.

Later that night, while Jake snored quietly beside me and Lucas breathed softly in the bassinet, I stared at the ceiling and replayed it all in my mind.

David's words. David's gaze. The warmth of the wine. The ease of the conversation. The part of me that came alive in that moment. The part I thought I'd lost.

And then the other part. The one I didn't want to look at too closely.

I'd broken my sobriety. I'd let one evening erase ten months of progress, because I wanted to feel like more than a mother. Because I wanted to feel wanted.

The guilt settled in, low and steady. But it wasn't loud enough to drown out the other feeling: the memory of being seen. Of being interesting. Desirable.

Jake hadn't looked at me like that in months. Maybe longer. I wanted to believe it was just the wine. That the moment would pass and everything would go back to normal. But deep down, I knew the truth. I was already looking forward to seeing David again.

Despite the guilt. Despite the promise. Despite everything I stood to lose.

The next week, I was surprised to see David in the coffee shop near my office during lunch. "Emily!" he called out, waving me over. "What a coincidence. I was just thinking about you." He seemed genuinely pleased to see me, but something about finding him at the exact place I always grabbed lunch felt... intentional. I didn't put too much thought into it back then.

The Thursday drinks became routine before I even realized I was counting on them. Every week, around five-thirty, David would pop his head into my office, and we'd wrap up whatever we were working on. Then we'd head down the street to Cellar Door for what we jokingly called "decompression therapy."

Each week, I told myself I'd stick to coffee or sparkling water. Every time, I ordered wine instead.

It was easy to rationalize. One evening a week didn't count. I was still mostly sober. I wasn't falling apart. I was just managing stress the way any working parent might.

"It's about boundaries," David said one Thursday, swirling the wine in his glass as we settled into our usual corner table. "If you don't separate work from home, everything bleeds together. And then you're mediocre at both."

"Speaking from experience?" I asked, letting the wine warm my throat and enjoying the way he always seemed to look straight through the noise in my head.

"Absolutely. I brought home stress into work, and work stress home. Eventually, I was miserable everywhere. Now I draw lines. I have times for thinking about things, and times for letting it go.

"This," he lifted his glass, "is one of those times."

"To proper compartmentalization," I said, raising mine.

As the weeks went on, our conversations shifted. Less about deadlines and meetings, more about everything else. His complicated family history, my fears about losing myself in motherhood, the way time felt different after kids. How identity faded under the weight of obligation.

He talked about wanting to move to Europe someday. I told him I sometimes fantasized about starting over somewhere no one knew me. We both pretended not to notice how often our knees bumped under the table, or how his hand would graze mine when he passed the wine.

"It changes after kids," David said once, after I'd confessed how far Jake and I had drifted. "The pressure either pulls you closer or pulls you apart."

"How do you know which one's happening?" I asked.

He looked at me for a long time. "You probably already do."

I didn't answer, but the words stayed with me. So did the way he said them. Quiet, certain, not unkind. I wasn't ready to admit anything out loud, but with David, I could almost imagine being someone brave enough to.

Wine made that easier too. I wasn't drinking like I used to, but on Thursdays, I came close. Two glasses turned into three, and by the time I got home, I was always a little unsteady. Never falling-down drunk, just loose enough to remember what it felt like to let go.

Jake noticed, in his way.

"You seem happier lately," he said one night, brushing his teeth while I changed into pajamas.

"Do I?" I asked, careful not to move too fast.

"Yeah. You seem more like yourself. Less... overwhelmed."

"Maybe I'm figuring it out," I said, sliding into bed beside him, hoping he wouldn't catch the scent of wine in my hair or on my breath.

He reached for my hand. "I'm really glad," he said. "I was worried for a while."

The guilt landed sharp and fast. He believed I was getting better. He thought my late nights were work stress or adjustment. He didn't know I was spending them with someone who made me feel seen in a way that was dangerously easy to crave.

"I love you," I said quietly.

"I love you too," he replied. There was a softness in his voice, maybe even relief.

And I meant it. I did. I loved Jake. I loved our children. I loved the life we were building.

But I also loved how David looked at me like I mattered. Like I was interesting. Like I was still a woman with something to say, not just someone holding everything together.

I told myself it was just the wine. Just friendship. Just the relief of being reminded that there was still a version of me underneath all of this who wasn't completely lost.

And for now, that was enough to keep going back.

Mostly, I loved how wine tasted when I was drinking it with someone who reminded me of who I used to be. Even if it meant betraying the promise I'd made to become the woman I was trying so hard to be.

The kiss happened on a Thursday evening in June, after one of those weeks that felt like it might never end. Lucas hadn't slept more than two hours at a time. Emma was in the middle of a clingy phase that made leaving for work feel like a daily heartbreak. And Jake had just told me about another last-minute business trip. The third in as many months right when I'd started to believe we might get a weekend together as a family.

"You look like you need something stronger than wine," David said as I walked into Cellar Door and sank into the seat across from him.

"I need a vacation," I muttered. "Or a nanny. Or a time machine that takes me back to when my biggest stress was project deadlines and not whether everyone ate a vegetable at dinner."

He signaled the waitress. "I can't offer time travel, but I can make tonight better than usual."

He ordered us cocktails, vodka-based, citrusy, deceptively light. Stronger than wine, smoother than I expected. It tasted like a break. Like possibility.

We talked about work frustrations, home chaos, and the usual things. But everything felt looser under the alcohol, like our problems had weight but could still be picked up and moved around. Like there might be space between the stress to breathe.

"You know what I admire about you?" David said, after we'd moved from cocktails back to wine.

"What?"

"You're not giving up. You're fighting for yourself. Most people let motherhood swallow them whole. You're trying to keep some part of you intact. That takes guts."

No one had ever said that to me before.

Jake told me I needed to "give it time." My mother called it a phase. Friends reassured me I'd "adjust eventually." No one had framed it as courage. Not until now.

"Thank you," I said, surprised by how unsteady my voice sounded.

"For what?"

"For getting it. For seeing me. For not making me feel like I'm just being dramatic or selfish."

"You're not," he said simply, reaching across the table and taking my hand. "You're just being honest."

Later, he walked me to my car, and we lingered there longer than made sense. The summer air was soft. The streetlights gave everything a gentle blur. I didn't want the night to end.

"I should go," I said, even though I hadn't moved.

"You should," he said, but stepped closer instead.

When he kissed me, I didn't stop him. I didn't even hesitate.

It wasn't a surprise. It felt like the answer to a question I hadn't let myself ask. His lips were warm, and he tasted like the wine we'd shared and the version of me I missed. For half a minute, I forgot about laundry and diapers and daycare emails. I was just a woman being kissed.

Then I remembered everything.

"I can't," I said, stepping back and reaching for my keys with hands that didn't feel steady.

"Emily..."

"I'm married. I have kids. I can't do this."

"I know," he said softly. "I'm not asking you to do anything you don't want to."

But that was the problem. I did want to. I wanted to feel seen, wanted, interesting. I wanted to keep talking with someone who thought I was brave instead of broken. I wanted a life that didn't need alcohol to feel manageable.

"This can't happen again," I said, sliding into the driver's seat before the pull got any stronger.

"It doesn't have to," David said, leaning down to my open window. "But, Emily... you deserve to be happy. However that looks."

On the way home, I replayed everything. his hand in mine, the kiss, the way he looked at me like I was still in there somewhere beneath the exhaustion. I thought about what it meant to survive a life, and what it meant to actually live one.

And I wondered when I'd stopped knowing the difference.

When I got home, Jake fell asleep on the couch. A business report was open across his chest. The lights were dim. The house was quiet. Both babies were sleeping soundly in their rooms. Nothing was out of place.

It was everything I'd asked for. Everything we'd built toward. So why did walking away from David's kiss feel harder than anything I'd done in years?

I poured a glass of wine from the bottle I hid in the closet. I needed something to make sense of the ache in my chest. I sat at the kitchen table, staring into the darkened living room, trying to untangle the contradictions that had become my life.

I loved Jake. I loved our kids. I loved the life we'd made on paper, at least. But I also loved how I felt on Thursday nights, sitting across from David in that dim wine bar, remembering what it was like to be seen. To feel like more than the default parent, the one who held everything together. To feel like someone worth watching, worth listening to, worth touching.

The wine didn't give me clarity, but it dulled the guilt just enough for the truth to surface: those Thursday nights had started to matter more than they should. More than anything else, really.

That meant something. Something important. Something I hadn't been ready to name until now. It meant I was in trouble. It meant I wasn't just missing who I used to be. I was chasing her down. And it meant I was probably going to kiss him again, no matter what I told myself about promises or boundaries or doing better.

I finished the wine and walked quietly upstairs. I checked on Emma first. She was curled around her stuffed bunny, breathing softly, one hand resting on the edge of her blanket. Lucas was sprawled in his crib, arms above his head, completely at peace.

They were beautiful. Pure. Innocent in ways I hadn't been in a long time. They deserved a mother who was steady. Present. Focused. They didn't deserve someone standing in the dark thinking about another man's lips.

I stood there for a long time, then made a decision I wanted to believe was final: I would end it. Whatever "it" was. I'd draw the line before it became something I couldn't come back from. I'd be the woman I'd promised to be. The one my family needed.

That resolve lasted exactly seven days.

The following Thursday, David appeared in my doorway at five-thirty, just like always. Same relaxed smile. Same quiet confidence. Same pulse of something dangerous and familiar in my chest.

"Ready for decompression therapy?" he asked.

I hesitated, gripping the edge of my desk like it might anchor me. "Actually, I think I should head home tonight. Be with the kids."

He nodded easily, like he'd already predicted the shift. "Of course. Rain check?"

"Rain check," I said, and I meant it for about ten minutes.

I made it all the way to the parking garage before turning around.

"David," I called as he stood waiting for the elevator.

He turned, and the look on his face said he'd known I'd come back.

"Change your mind?"

"I think I need that drink after all."

"I was hoping you'd say that."

Later, when he kissed me goodbye, I didn't flinch. I didn't apologize. I didn't explain.

I kissed him back. Fully. Intentionally.

And on the way home, I wasn't thinking about the promises I'd broken or the damage I might do. I just knew something had shifted and I wasn't sure I wanted to stop it.

Chapter Six

Everything Falls Apart

After that kiss, something shifted in me.

It wasn't an earthquake. It didn't flip a switch overnight. It was slower than that. Like water heating on the stove, just a few degrees at a time, until suddenly it's boiling, and you don't know how it got there.

David and I kept texting first about work, harmless things. But then came the personal updates, the late-night check-ins, the flirty comments we pretended not to take seriously. Every Thursday night drink stretched later. Conversations turned deeper. The pull between us was impossible to ignore.

For that first month, he was everything I needed him to be. Attentive without being pushy. Curious without pressing too hard. He listened, really listened, in a way that felt rare. When he shared stories about himself, it didn't feel like bait. It felt like an invitation. And when we kissed, there was no pressure. Just two people giving into something that had been building for weeks.

"You make me feel like myself again," I told him one warm evening in June. I meant every word.

"Good," he whispered, fingers sliding through my hair. "You deserve to feel alive."

I clung to that. To the way he saw me. Not as a mother or a wife or someone trying to stay afloat but as someone who was beautiful and still worth wanting. Still capable of being chosen. The guilt was there, but I could tuck it away. Feeling seen after years of fading into the background made the risk feel worth it.

But as summer crept on, David's attention started to tighten around me. At first, it felt like flattery. The texts came more often, not just during the day but in the evenings, when he knew I was home with Jake and the kids.

"Thinking of you," he'd sent while I was running baths.

"Missing your smile," while Jake grilled burgers and the kids chased each other around the backyard.

"Can't wait to see you again," pinging through during Saturday morning pancakes.

At first, it felt romantic. Like I had this secret admirer following me through my messy domestic life, reaching for me across the chaos. But then it started feeling less like affection and more like demand. He wanted my attention. Constantly, he needed reassurance that I wasn't drifting away.

"Why didn't you answer my text?" he asked one Thursday.

"I was putting the kids to bed," I told him. "I can't always respond right away."

"I just worry when I don't hear from you," he said. Something in his voice had sharpened. "You matter too much to me."

He started asking how I was spending my weekends. Making comments about Jake that sounded casual but always left a bruise. He planted doubt with subtle precision.

"Does he even notice when you're upset?" he asked once, after I'd mentioned Jake forgetting to take out the trash again.

"He notices," I said, though I wasn't so sure anymore.

"The woman I see deserves better," David said. "Someone who puts her first."

I didn't realize it then, but he was carving out a narrative. Him and me on one side and Jake on the other. I was too caught up in the rush to see it for what it was. Manipulation wrapped in affection.

The more tangled things got with David, the more I turned back to wine. A glass before meeting him to calm the guilt. Another during dinner, to take the edge off his questions. And more when I got home, to silence the voice in my head asking what the hell I was doing.

That's when Jake noticed.

I was in the kitchen one night in July, glass in hand, sliding dishes into the dishwasher. Jake appeared in the doorway and just stood there, watching me. I didn't have to look up to know something had shifted in his face.

"Emily," he said, low and steady. "You're drinking again."

I froze, wine sloshing in the glass. "What do you mean?"

"I mean there's an open bottle on the counter and that's not your first glass." His voice was calm, but heavy. "You promised me. You poured it all out. You said you were done."

My heart started thudding. "It's just a glass with dinner."

"It's not just one glass. I know the signs. Your eyes. Your voice. Emily, come on."

I wanted to argue, but nothing I could say would make this better. The truth was ugly, and it sat between us like a third person. I wasn't drinking because of stress at work or the kids. I was drinking because I was lying to my husband and sneaking around with another man.

"I've been stressed," I said finally. "You've been traveling. It's just been a lot."

Jake didn't raise his voice. His face softened. That made it worse.

"Then talk to me," he said. "Don't go back to this. Don't make me live through that version of you again."

I remembered that version too. The nights we dumped bottles down the sink. The promises I made, crying on the floor. Back then, I was desperate to fix things. This version of me wasn't desperate to fix anything. She was desperate to hide.

"I'm fine," I said. "This isn't like before."

"That's what you said before," he replied. "And then it was."

He took the glass from my hand gently. "Look at me."

I did, trying to steady my body, trying to keep my voice level.

"Your eyes are glassy," he said. "You're swaying. You're drunk, Emily. Our kids are upstairs getting ready for bed."

His words hit like a slap. Not because they were cruel, but because they were true. I had no defense. Not one.

"I thought you were getting better," he said, his voice cracking. "I thought you were okay."

I wanted to scream that I was better, that I had been happier, that someone had made me feel alive again. But I couldn't say any of that, because that someone wasn't him.

"I am okay," I whispered. "I'm just... figuring things out."

Jake stared at me for a long time, like he was trying to see the version of me he used to believe in.

But while Jake was worried about the wine, David was pushing harder.

"You've been different," David said one night on the phone. "Distant. Are you pulling away from me?"

"I'm just overwhelmed," I said. "Trying to keep everything together."

"Balance?" he scoffed. "What we have shouldn't need balancing. It should be everything."

"I have a family," I said.

"And they don't appreciate you," he snapped. "You deserve someone who sees you, Emily."

When he started talking about my children, I finally snapped.

"Don't talk about them like that."

"I'm just saying they deserve a mother who doesn't drink herself to sleep every night."

His words landed with a thud. Because he wasn't wrong. Not completely. The drinking was getting harder to hide.

"How do you even know?" I asked.

"I see it. I smell it. You think I don't notice?"

And that's when I realized what had changed. David wasn't just my escape anymore. He was watching me. Monitoring me. Keeping tabs.

"Maybe I need to cut back," I muttered.

"Or maybe," he said, "you need to leave him and be with someone who actually loves you."

And just like that, I knew I was standing at the edge of a cliff. One step forward and everything would fall.

By August, the wine was a daily ritual. Not just on Thursdays. Not just before seeing David. I drank before he called, during our conversations when his voice curled through the phone at the worst possible times, and afterward, especially afterward, when the shame caught up to me and I needed to drown it out.

"You seem different lately," Jake said one evening as I poured my third glass of wine at the dinner table.

"Different how?" I asked, sharper than I meant to.

"Anxious. Distracted. Like you're always bracing for something."

He wasn't wrong. I was. David had started appearing in places he shouldn't have been casually, like it was nothing. He showed up at the coffee shop near my office. At the park where I took the kids. Once at the grocery store. Always with a shrug and a smile. "Just in the neighborhood."

I took a long sip, feeling the sting in the back of my throat.

"Just work stress," I muttered.

"Maybe you should talk to someone," Jake said gently. "A counselor or..."

"I don't need a counselor," I snapped. "I need you to stop analyzing everything I do."

He didn't push. He just looked at me with that wounded expression that used to get to me when I still felt like I deserved his concern. But by then, I felt like I was trapped in a house with two men watching my every move.

One with quiet disappointment. The other with obsession.

The day it all came to a head was one of those soft, early fall Saturdays. I took the kids to the park, hoping for a moment of peace. Emma on the swings, Lucas in the sandbox, sunshine warming the back of my neck. Just us. Just a normal afternoon.

And then I heard his voice.

"Emily."

I turned, and there he was. David. Standing too close, wearing jeans and a button-down like he'd dressed to be seen. No running gear. No excuse.

"What are you doing here?" I whispered.

"Saw you on my run," he said. A lie so flimsy it made my stomach flip.

"Not here. Not in front of them."

"When then?" His tone was all too familiar. Urgent, emotional, demanding. "You've been ignoring me."

"David, please. Please. Just go."

But he didn't. He stepped closer, his voice low and sharp. "I'm tired of being your secret. I'm tired of watching you go home to him."

"Mommy," Emma called from the swing. "Who's that man?"

"Just someone from work, sweetheart," I said, forcing a smile while my insides scrambled. "Keep playing."

"You need to choose," David said. "Him or me. This in-between is killing me."

"Not now."

"What if I told him?" His eyes narrowed. "What if I called Jake and told him everything?"

My blood ran cold. "David, are you serious? You wouldn't."

He tilted his head. "Maybe it's time the truth came out. Maybe it's time everyone knew."

I took a step back. "You're scaring me."

"Good," he said. "Maybe that's what it takes."

"Mommy, can we go to the monkey bars?" Emma came running over, all smiles and innocence.

David crouched slightly, looking at my daughter like he belonged there. "You must be Emma. Your mom talks about you all the time."

"Don't," I said, stepping between them. "Don't talk to my children."

"Why not? If we're going to be together..."

"We're not." My voice cracked. "We're not anything anymore."

I grabbed Emma's hand and put Lucas into his stroller. "We're leaving."

David's voice followed me as I walked away. "This isn't over. I'll be in touch."

That night, after the kids were asleep, I sat at the kitchen table with a bottle of wine and tried to make sense of what my life had become. The affair that once made me feel seen and alive now made me feel hunted. I wasn't even sure who I was hiding from anymore. Jake, David, myself?

My phone buzzed on the table. Another message from David.

"I meant what I said. Choose."

I poured another glass. I had no idea how to fix any of it.

The next two weeks were a blur of nerves and wine. David started calling my office line directly. Sent flowers I had to hide in the break room trash. Left voicemails laced with longing and fury. And then, he started following me.

At first, I told myself I was imagining it. But when I saw his car behind mine three days in a row, it became undeniable.

When I finally confronted him, he didn't even try to deny it.

"I just wanted to see where you live," he said, like that made it okay. "I want to understand your whole life."

"This is stalking," I told him, my voice shaking. "You're stalking me. Please stop David"

"Stalking? Are you serious? "I'm loving you," he said.

I wanted to scream. I wanted to confess everything to Jake, burn it all down, and start over. But I did what I'd been doing all along. I went home, poured another glass, and tried to pretend I still had control.

David's threats, his presence, the constant buzz of fear. I drank to quiet it all. I drank to forget the version of me I'd become. And when the wine hit, for just a moment, I could believe none of it was real.

But it was. And it was closing in fast.

It ended on a Monday evening in October.

I was stirring a pot of pasta on the stove, half-listening to Emma and Lucas giggling over some cartoon in the living room. The kitchen smelled like garlic and butter, and for a brief second, everything felt almost normal if I didn't think too hard. Jake was due back from a work trip that night, and I was quietly relieved at the thought of another adult finally being in the house. I needed backup. I needed someone to help me feel like the floor wasn't crumbling beneath my feet.

Then the doorbell rang.

I wiped my hands on a dish towel and glanced through the peephole.

David.

Standing on my front porch, clutching a manila envelope like it held my entire life inside it.

My stomach dropped. He'd never come to my house before. Never crossed that line.

I cracked the door just enough to speak, my voice tight. "What the hell are you doing here?"

"I called. You didn't answer." His eyes were wild, unsteady, and needy. The kind of desperation that makes your skin crawl.

"You need to leave. My kids are inside."

"Then come out here. Just for a minute. We need to talk."

"No," I said, sharper this time. "You can't be here. Not now. Not ever."

He held the envelope higher, like it was proof of something. "I printed everything. Our messages, the emails. I was going to give it all to Jake myself, but I figured I'd let you come clean first."

I stared at him, the air thick in my lungs. "Come clean?"

"Leave him, Emily. Be with me. You said it yourself. We belong together."

"There is no us," I said, my voice as steady as I could make it. "There never was. This was a mistake. It's over."

His expression darkened. "It's not over until I say it is."

That's when Jake's car turned into the driveway.

Panic lit up my chest. "Shit."

I stepped outside, closing the door behind me just as Jake pulled in. He stepped out of the car, saw David, and his face shifted. First confusion, then concern, then something colder.

"Emily?" he called. "What's going on?"

David turned to greet him like it was all perfectly normal. "You must be Jake. I'm David Blake. I work with Emily."

Jake's eyes flicked to me, then back to David. "Is there a problem here?"

"Actually, yes," David said, voice calm but dangerous. "I think you should know what your wife's been up to."

"Stop." My voice cracked. "David, don't."

Jake didn't need to hear more. The envelope, my pleading, the history written all over our faces. He saw it.

"Get off my property," Jake said, quiet but firm.

"You don't want to hear what I have to say?" David asked, smug, like he thought he was doing Jake a favor.

Jake didn't even blink. "Leave. Or I'm calling the cops."

David hesitated for a beat too long.

Jake pulled out his phone. "Nine-one-one, what's your emergency?"

David looked from the phone to Jake, then to me, shrinking in the doorway. "This isn't over," he said.

"Yes, it is," Jake answered.

David tossed the envelope to Jake and walked away.

Jake bent down, picked it up, and held it out to me without opening it. "Inside. Now."

The fight that followed cracked something deep inside me.

He didn't even read the papers. He didn't have to. My guilt was in the air between us, thick and sour. The way I'd begged David, the panicked look on my face, the way Jake had watched it all unfold like a slow-motion car crash.

"You've been having an affair," Jake said. It wasn't a question.

I nodded. What else could I do?

He shook his head, stunned. "How long has he been following you?"

"A few weeks."

"You didn't think I should know that? You didn't think it mattered that a man was stalking my wife and showing up where my kids play?"

"I thought I could handle it."

"By drinking every night? By lying to me and putting our family at risk?"

He wasn't yelling. That almost made it worse.

That night, Jake called the police himself. Filed the complaint. David was gone within two days, fired from the company, and slapped with a restraining order.

But the damage between us? That stayed.

"I can't trust you," Jake said the next night, after the kids were asleep. "Not just because of the affair. Because you were scared and you still didn't tell me. You drank instead. You gambled with our safety."

"I was scared," I whispered.

"You should've been," he said. "But you should've been scared enough to tell the truth. Not numb it away."

And with that, I knew this wasn't just the end of an affair. This was the beginning of losing everything.

In the days after everything exploded, I did what I could to prove to Jake that David was gone. Completely, irreversibly gone. The restraining order had already been filed, but I went further. I blocked

David's number, deleted every text, every email, and every photo. I scrubbed my phone like I was trying to erase a crime scene. I even rearranged my work schedule so I wouldn't risk running into any colleagues who might bring up his name by accident.

Three days after the order was filed, David tried to contact me through someone at work. I didn't hesitate. I reported it to the police immediately. I wanted Jake to see I was taking this seriously, that I understood, finally, what I had let into our lives.

"He's gone," I told Jake one night, laying the paperwork out on the kitchen table. Police reports. Call logs. Screenshots showing the blocked numbers and deleted accounts. "There's no way he can reach me now."

Jake looked at the papers, then looked at me.

"That's not the point," he said quietly. "The point is, you let it get that far. You had an affair with a man who became dangerous, and instead of protecting this family, you tried to manage it yourself with lies and alcohol."

I opened my mouth to argue to tell him I didn't know David would spiral like this, that it had started as something light, a distraction, a way to feel like myself again. But I couldn't say it. Not with Jake sitting across from me, shoulders slumped like the weight of it all had finally cracked something inside him. Not with my own shame sitting right there beside the empty wineglass in front of me.

"I ended it the moment I realized what he was," I said.

Jake shook his head. "No. You ended it when he threatened your family. When he showed up at our front door. When he forced your hand. Emily, you've been drinking every night for months. You've been lying to me for longer than that. You put the kids in danger, and you didn't say a word."

That landed like a punch. I'd justified so much to myself. I told myself I could fix it. I told myself the wine helped me stay calm, helped me stay functional. But I wasn't calm. And I wasn't functional. I was spiraling.

"I can change," I said. "I'll stop drinking. I'll go to counseling. I'll do whatever it takes."

"You could've done that before," Jake said, not unkindly. "I asked you to. I begged you."

"Please don't give up on us."

He looked at me for a long time. And then he said, softly, "I'm not giving up on you. But I am giving up on this marriage. I can't do it anymore."

Two weeks later, he made it official.

"This is over," he said, standing in the doorway with his car keys in one hand and a custody agreement in the other. "I'm filing for divorce. And I'm asking for full custody. You're not safe to be around them right now."

I couldn't breathe. "Please don't take my children."

"I'm not taking them," he said, and his voice cracked. "You gave them up the moment you picked wine and a man like that over their safety."

I didn't have anything left to say.

He turned away and started walking upstairs. "You should call your parents," he added over his shoulder. "You're going to need support."

"Jake..." I reached for him, but he didn't stop. He didn't yell. He didn't slam the door. He just left the room.

"I can't save you from yourself," he said. "And I won't let you take the kids down with you."

Then, he was gone.

The house went still.

The wine glass on the table hadn't moved. Neither had I.

Cartoons were still playing in the other room.

The sound of my family moving on without me was deafening.

That weekend, I stood in the hallway and watched Jake pack up our life in cardboard boxes. The kids' things. The car seats. Emma's pink dresser. Lucas's fire truck blanket. Bit by bit, my family was being carried out the front door.

"Are we moving?" Emma asked, watching her dad haul her stuffed animals out to the car.

"Daddy's taking you to Grandma and Grandpa's for a little while," I said, trying to keep my voice steady.

"What about you?"

"I need to stay here and... fix some things."

"What kind of things?"

How do you tell your daughter the truth? That you broke everything good. That you drank and lied and brought a dangerous man into your lives because you couldn't face your own loneliness.

"Just... grown-up things," I said. "But I'll see you soon."

"Promise?"

I nodded. "Promise."

She looked at me like she wasn't sure if she believed me anymore.

Lucas didn't say much. He just clung to my neck when Jake tried to carry him outside.

"Mama stay," he whispered.

"I have to stay," I told him, my voice breaking. "But Daddy's going to take really good care of you, okay?"

Jake found me in the kitchen, hands wrapped around a coffee mug I'd filled but hadn't touched.

"This doesn't have to be permanent," he said. "If you get help, real help, and stay sober, we can talk about it."

"How long?"

"I don't know. A year. Maybe longer. As long as it takes to trust that the change is real."

A year. Without my children. Without Jake. Without the life I'd already lost but hadn't admitted to yet.

"I love you," I said.

"I love you too," he said. "That's why I have to do this."

He kissed me on the forehead. It wasn't angry. It wasn't warm, either. It was... final.

Emma ran back to me for one last hug. "I'll miss you, Mommy."

"I'll miss you too, sweetheart. Be good for Daddy."

"I will. And get better, okay?"

I nodded. I couldn't speak.

Lucas gave me a sticky kiss on the cheek and toddled off after his sister, already excited by the promise of something new.

I stood in the driveway and watched the car pull away.

The silence afterward was unbearable.

Inside, I went straight to the pantry. I pulled out the bottle I'd hidden the week before—just in case.

Just one glass, I told myself.

Just enough to take the edge off.

One glass became two. Then the bottle was empty.

The next morning, I woke up on the kitchen floor. Still in yesterday's clothes. My head pounding. My mouth dry. My family gone.

And the only thing left?

The wine.

Jake had been right. I wasn't going to stop. I was already telling myself I needed it. Already negotiating with the monster I thought I'd outrun.

This was the beginning of something darker. Something lonelier.

For the first time, I was truly alone with it.

And I knew I hadn't hit rock bottom yet. But I was close. So close.

You've reached the midpoint of *From Wine Mom To Sober Mom*.

Thank you for coming this far with me. There are still plenty of twists, honest moments, and stories left in the rest of the book, and I hope you'll stick around for the journey ahead.

Before you dive back in, I just wanted to pause for a moment and ask: if you're finding the book meaningful so far, would you consider leaving a quick, honest review on Amazon? Even a few sentences can help new readers find the story and makes a big difference for indie authors like me.

Amazon Link for Your Review

https://www.amazon.com/dp/B0FN8KP8X8

Thank you for reading and now, on to the rest of the story!

Chapter Seven

Winning the Battle, Losing the War

THREE MONTHS AFTER JAKE left with the kids, I found myself sitting in a family court waiting room, doing my best impression of a mother who had her life together.

The truth? I'd had two glasses of wine with breakfast. Just enough to keep the panic at bay. Just enough to function.

The room buzzed under fluorescent lights. Beige walls, plastic chairs. Everyone sat stiffly, scrolling through phones or staring ahead, waiting to have their family lives dissected and turned into court filings and custody schedules.

A young woman with a clipboard approached. "Emily Matthews?"

I stood too fast. The floor swayed for half a second.

"I'm Jennifer Walsh," she said. "Your attorney for today."

"Thanks," I said, trying to sound steady. "I'm ready."

She paused, eyeing me. "You sure you're okay? You look a little... tense."

"Just nervous a bit," I said. "First time doing anything like this."

She nodded and motioned toward the hallway. "Fair warning. This might be rougher than I anticipated. Jake's lawyer is leaning hard on the David Blake situation and your drinking. But we've got some solid ground too."

My stomach sank. "Like what?"

"Well, for starters, you were the victim in the Blake situation, not the aggressor. You went to the police. Got a restraining order. That's proof you acted to protect your kids once you realized the danger."

We walked into the conference room. Jake was already seated with his attorney, a woman in her fifties who looked like she'd trained her whole life for moments like this.

"And second," Jennifer whispered as we sat down, "Jake's travel schedule is well documented. He's been gone, on average, half the month every month for two years. Courts care about consistency. Especially for kids this young."

The mediator, Mrs. Rodriguez, called things to order. She had the kind of soft, worn face that looked like it had absorbed a hundred versions of this same conversation.

"We'll begin with custody," she said. "Mr. Matthews, you're requesting primary physical custody of the children?"

Jake's lawyer jumped in. "Yes, Your Honor. Mr. Matthews has deep concerns about Mrs. Matthews' ability to maintain a stable home. There are clear issues with alcohol and poor judgment, specifically her relationship with a man who later stalked her family."

Mrs. Rodriguez turned to me. "Mrs. Matthews, how do you respond?"

I took a breath, feeling the wine settle just enough to keep my hands from shaking. "I've made mistakes. I'll own that. But I've always been the one who takes care of Emma and Lucas. I know their schedules, their schools, their routines. Jake's job keeps him traveling. He's gone nearly half the month."

Jake's lawyer opened a folder. "We'd like to submit documentation of Mrs. Matthews' involvement with David Blake, a man who ultimately harassed and threatened her family."

"Objection," Jennifer cut in. "The record shows Mrs. Matthews was the one who took legal action to protect her children. She filed a police report and secured a restraining order. Mr. Blake has since moved out of state and poses no ongoing threat."

Mrs. Rodriguez flipped through the documents. "Mrs. Matthews, can you walk me through that timeline?"

I stuck to the script we'd practiced. "It started as a workplace relationship. I ended it as soon as his behavior became alarming. When he started showing up around my children, I went to the police. I haven't had contact with him since the restraining order was issued."

Mrs. Rodriguez looked up. "And the concerns about alcohol?"

This was the part I'd been dreading. "I've had drinks, yes. But not to the extent being claimed. I'm a working mother navigating a painful divorce. My drinking has stayed within normal limits."

Jake's lawyer wasn't satisfied. "Your Honor, we believe the drinking has been excessive."

"Any DUIs? ER visits? CPS reports? Issues raised by teachers or childcare providers?" Mrs. Rodriguez asked.

"No, Your Honor," Jake's lawyer said. "But..."

"Mr. Matthews," she said, turning to Jake. "During your marriage, did you ever witness your wife endanger the children while under the influence?"

Jake hesitated. "No. But she was often tired. Sometimes her speech seemed slurred. I was worried."

"Was there ever any formal intervention or reported incident?"

"No."

Mrs. Rodriguez nodded, taking notes. "Your travel records indicate you were gone 182 days last year. How will you manage full-time parenting with that schedule?"

"I can figure something out with my company," Jake said. "More local. I'm willing to cut back."

"That's good," she said, "but courts typically view post-separation career changes as temporary adjustments, not proof of long-term consistency."

She turned to Jennifer and me. "Mrs. Matthews has maintained steady employment and primary caregiving throughout the children's lives."

Jennifer leaned in close. "You're holding steady," she whispered. "This is good."

Jake's attorney shifted tactics. "Your Honor, we're also concerned about Mrs. Matthews' judgment in romantic relationships. The David Blake incident put her children at risk."

"She took immediate action," Mrs. Rodriguez said calmly. "She ended the relationship and pursued legal protection. Adults make poor romantic choices. It only becomes relevant if they don't act to safeguard their children, which Mrs. Matthews clearly did."

We spent another two hours in that room, parsing through school zoning, shared holidays, bedtime routines.

Finally, the mediator laid her pen down. "Based on the testimony and documentation, Mrs. Matthews will retain primary physical custody of Emma and Lucas. Mr. Matthews will have parenting time every other weekend and one evening per week. This reflects the historical caregiving arrangement and prioritizes the children's need for stability during this transition."

I'd won.

Despite the drinking, despite David, despite the chaos of the past year. I still walked out of there with my kids.

Outside the courthouse, Jennifer gave me a look that bordered on impressed.

"You did well in there," she said. "Jake's side was clearly ready to push harder, but they didn't have the evidence. We held our ground."

"What happens now?" I asked.

"Now you show the court they were right to trust you. Keep the house stable. Keep childcare consistent. And document everything. Texts, calendars, expenses. Jake's not going to let this go. He'll be looking for a reason to reopen the case."

I nodded.

I had what I asked for. What I fought for. What I told myself I needed.

But I knew even then that this wasn't the end of the story.

It was just the next round in a battle I was still losing.

That evening, I celebrated with a bottle of champagne.

I told myself it was to mark a milestone. I'd won custody. I'd outmaneuvered Jake. I'd proved something to him, to the court, to myself.

I didn't call it what it really was: relief in liquid form. Relief that I hadn't lost my children. Relief that I could still look like a capable mother, even if I didn't always feel like one.

The kids came back the next week.

Emma ran into my arms as soon as she saw me, holding on like she wasn't sure I was real. Lucas buried his face in my shoulder and wouldn't let go for most of the day.

"I missed you so much," Emma said.

"I missed you too, sweetheart," I told her. "But we're together now. Everything's going to be okay."

And I meant it. In that moment, I believed I could do this. That I could be enough. That I could rebuild what I'd nearly lost.

The first week felt like a second chance. I took time off work and focused entirely on the kids. We had movie nights and pancake breakfasts. I let them sleep in my bed when they needed extra reassurance. I didn't drink during the day. I waited until after they were asleep, and even then, just a glass or two. Enough to take the edge off, nothing more.

But the second week was harder.

Emma started waking up from nightmares, asking if Daddy was coming back to take her away. Lucas became clingy, crying when I left him at daycare, crying when I picked him up, crying just without any apparent reason. He didn't have the words to explain what he was feeling, and I didn't always have the patience to figure it out.

That's when I started pouring earlier.

A glass while making dinner, because the whining was constant. A glass in the afternoon on weekends, when both kids were melting down and the house was a mess. I told myself it was just a little help, just something to smooth the edges of long, demanding days.

Then came the weekdays. A glass after school drop-off. A quick sip while folding laundry. A refill while writing emails for work.

I wasn't getting drunk. Not really. I was managing. Still getting everything done. Still packing lunches and brushing hair and showing up to parent-teacher meetings with a smile.

But I was unraveling.

The money ran tight faster than I expected. Our house had made sense when Jake and I shared the bills. Alone, it was suffocating. Childcare, groceries, utilities, legal fees. Everything added up until I couldn't breathe.

One night I sat at the kitchen table surrounded by unpaid bills. My stomach clenched as I looked at the numbers. No matter how I rearranged them, they didn't make sense.

"We're going to have to move," I told Emma that evening.

She looked up from her coloring book. "Move where?"

"Somewhere smaller. An apartment. Just for a little while."

Her face fell. "But this is our house."

"I know," I said. "But sometimes grown-ups have to make hard choices."

What I didn't tell her was that I'd already looked at apartments I could afford, and most were in neighborhoods with schools that made me nervous. What I didn't tell her was that the wine I bought to feel okay was eating into our grocery budget. What I didn't tell her was that some nights, after she and Lucas were asleep, I sat at that same kitchen table and seriously thought about calling Jake.

Not to fight. Not to ask for more money.

But to ask if he would take us back.

Because no matter how much I loved my children, no matter how hard I tried, I was starting to realize that loving them might not be enough to save us from me.

The apartment was a two-bedroom in a run-down complex that smelled faintly of mildew and stale carpet. Emma and Lucas would share a room. I'd sleep on a pullout couch in the living room.

The rent was manageable. Just over half of what our mortgage had been. But it felt like failure dressed up as practicality.

"It's cozy," I said, forcing a smile as we stepped into the empty space.

Emma looked around with a frown. "It's small."

She wasn't wrong.

"Sometimes small is better," I said. "Less to clean. Easier to keep warm. More time to spend together."

Lucas didn't seem to mind. At three and a half, he adjusted easily. Maybe too easily. Emma, now five, understood what this meant. Smaller apartment, tighter budget. Daddy had the house. Mommy didn't. The math added up in ways I couldn't explain away.

"Can we paint my room pink?" she asked.

"Of course we can," I said, already picturing the credit card balance.

Single parenting didn't leave much room to breathe. Every decision was mine. Every tantrum, every fever, every forgotten permission slip. There was no handoff. No "can you take this one?"

It was just me.

And the wine.

Jake stuck to the custody agreement. Every other weekend, Wednesday nights. He'd pull into the parking lot in his newer car, freshly shaved and well rested, and the kids would race toward him like he was Santa Claus.

"How's school going?" He'd ask Emma.

"Good," she'd say, even though I'd just gotten an email from her teacher about her slipping grades.

"Are you being good for Mommy?" he'd ask Lucas.

"Yes," Lucas would reply, even though he'd thrown his snack across the kitchen that morning and spent twenty minutes screaming on the floor.

Jake didn't stay long. He'd drop them off on Sunday evenings with polite detachment, like a courier returning a fragile package. The kids would be quieter those nights, adjusting back to life in our apartment with its mismatched furniture and ever-present undercurrent of tension.

By then, I was usually on my second glass of wine.

"Mommy, your eyes look tired," Emma said one night while I checked her math homework.

"I am tired," I said. "Being a mommy is hard work."

"Daddy says you should sleep more."

I looked up. "What else does Daddy say?"

She shrugged. "Just that we should be extra good for you because it's hard being a single mommy."

I knew what he was doing. He was planting seeds, gently shaping the narrative. Daddy as the steady one. Mommy as the struggling one.

That night, I poured myself another glass. Bigger this time.

By spring, drinking became part of my rhythm. Not to black out. Not even to feel drunk. Just to blur the noise. To soften the sharp edges of everything I was failing at. It worked until it didn't.

Jake started documenting.

I didn't catch on at first. He'd show up to pick up the kids and casually record video on his phone. Nothing overt. Just enough to capture my tone, my face, the way I moved or slurred a word if I wasn't careful.

He took photos of the kids standing in the kitchen. Photos that just happened to include a half-empty wine bottle on the counter. He noticed dishes piling up, laundry waiting to be folded, toys scattered in the corners.

One Wednesday, he paused before leaving.

"Are you feeling okay?" he asked. "You seem a little off."

"I'm fine," I said. I'd had two glasses with dinner. I was relaxed. I was happy to see my kids.

"Your speech is a little slow," he said, phone angled toward me. "Maybe you should talk to a doctor. See if there's something going on."

I smiled tightly. "Just tired."

But I knew what he was doing. And he knew I knew.

He wasn't going to argue. He was going to document. Quietly, methodically, like someone building a case.

He was getting ready to try again.

To take them.

And I should have been terrified. That should have been the wake-up call.

Instead, it just made me want another drink.

The incident that changed everything happened on a Thursday in June.

Emma reminded me about the school concert at breakfast. I'd forgotten, of course. Work had been hectic, the kind of day that drains you before it's even lunch. Then groceries with both kids, Lucas melting down in the cereal aisle, Emma asking for snacks we couldn't afford. By the time we got home, I was unraveling.

While making dinner, I poured a glass of wine. Just one, I told myself. It would help me reset. Help me be present for the concert. Patient for the excitement. Grounded, maybe.

One glass turned into two while Emma practiced her song in the living room. She was off-key but enthusiastic. I smiled and told her she sounded great.

Two glasses became three while I dug through the laundry, searching for something she could wear that didn't look like it had been crumpled under a pile of unfolded clothes.

By the time we had to leave, I knew I shouldn't drive. I wasn't stumbling or slurring, but I wasn't sober.

"Mommy, we need to go," Emma said, checking the clock with a quiet urgency that didn't belong in a six-year-old's voice.

"I know, sweetheart. Just give me a minute."

I stood in the kitchen, staring at the keys. I thought about not going. I could say I wasn't feeling well, that we'd go to the next one. There's always a next one.

But Emma had been practicing for weeks. Her teacher said all the parents would be there. She'd asked me to sit in the front row.

"I'm fine," I told her, keeping my voice steady. "Just a little sick. Maybe we should skip it tonight."

Her face fell. "But I practiced so hard."

That should've been enough to stop me. But I told her we'd go. I splashed cold water on my face and grabbed the keys, already halfway through rationalizing it. It wasn't far. I'd drive slowly. I'd be careful.

And I was. Ten miles under the speed limit, white-knuckled, hyper-aware of every stop sign, every pedestrian, every car. No music. Just Emma humming beside me, practicing her part.

We made it to the school. Barely.

Emma was radiant on stage. Confident, grinning, completely in her element. I sat in the second row, smiling like the other parents, clapping when she sang. I looked like everyone else. But inside, I felt sick. I wasn't thinking about the performance. I was thinking about the drive home, about how close I'd come to something irreversible.

Parents mingled after the concert. Small talk. Compliments.

"She's such a talented little girl," one mom said. "You must be so proud."

I nodded. "I am." And I meant it. But that pride was tangled up in guilt, fear, and shame. I tried not to breathe too close to anyone.

We got home. I put the kids to bed. They were happy. I should have been relieved.

But instead of taking that night for what it was. A line I'd crossed, a clear warning. I poured another glass. Just one more, to steady myself.

That's the part that sticks with me.

It wasn't the concert. It wasn't the drive. It was the moment I poured that glass afterward.

That's when I knew how far gone I really was.

Three days later, the police came to my door.

It was just after nine at night. The kids were asleep upstairs. I'd had a few glasses of wine enough to feel it but not enough, I thought, to raise alarm. I never found out exactly what triggered the welfare check. Maybe someone from school called Jake. Maybe he noticed something in the kids. Or maybe he'd simply decided it was time.

The officers were polite but firm. They asked to come inside, and said they needed to verify the children were safe. I let them in, heart pounding. Emma was tucked in with her favorite blanket. Lucas was snoring softly. They were fine.

But the officers still noted the wine bottles in the kitchen, the stale smell in the air, the mess in the living room. They noted the alcohol on my breath. One of them asked if I'd had anything to drink that evening. I said yes. Just a little.

Two weeks later, I was back in court. This time, no one was on my side.

"Your Honor," Jake's lawyer began, "we have documented evidence that Mrs. Matthews has created an unsafe environment for the children due to chronic alcohol use."

They had photos. Some I didn't know Jake had taken. Audio recordings. Notes from teachers. The police report.

"Mrs. Matthews," the judge said, "can you explain why police officers found you under the influence while supervising your children on the evening of June 15th?"

I tried to keep my voice steady. "I'd had a glass of wine with dinner."

"Do you believe that's appropriate given the circumstances of your custody arrangement?"

I wanted to say yes. I wanted to say it was normal. That I wasn't the only parent who drank a glass of wine after a long day. But I knew that answer wouldn't matter. Not now.

Then Jake's lawyer brought up the concert. Apparently, Emma's teacher had noticed something that night and was worried enough to report it.

I sat there listening to people discuss my drinking like it was a math problem. Measurable, documentable, black and white.

In the end, the judge didn't hesitate. Custody was transferred to Jake. I was given supervised visitation, contingent on completing an alcohol treatment program.

When I walked out of the courtroom, Emma and Lucas were sitting on a bench with Jake's mother. They didn't fully understand what had just happened.

"Are we going home with you?" Emma asked.

"Not today," I said. "You're going to stay with Daddy for a little while."

She blinked, confused. "How long is a little while?"

I didn't answer. I just told her I loved her. That none of this was her fault.

Lucas hugged my legs. "Mama sad?"

I nodded. "Yeah. Mama's sad."

I watched them leave with Jake. The same scene I'd lived before, but this time it felt final.

I drove back to the apartment and poured a glass of wine. I told myself it was just to cope with the day. Just one.

Within a month, I couldn't pay rent. Child support was suspended until I met court conditions. I lost my job after a series of late arrivals and early departures I couldn't explain away.

And I lost the illusion that I was still holding it together.

I'd won custody by looking stable on paper, but I couldn't live up to the image I'd created. The wine I used to manage the stress of parenting had made me unfit to do it at all.

Now, standing in an empty apartment, surrounded by half-packed boxes and unpaid bills, I finally saw what I hadn't wanted to admit.

This wasn't just a rough patch. This wasn't a bad season. I wasn't in control.

Rock bottom didn't look like a single dramatic moment. It looked like a quiet Monday in June. It looked like getting what you fought for and realizing you couldn't keep it. It looked like telling yourself it was just one glass until it wasn't.

Chapter Eight

When Your Body Says No

THREE MONTHS HAD PASSED since I lost custody of Emma and Lucas, and I woke up sprawled on the cold bathroom floor, my body convulsing as I vomited blood into the toilet.

The apartment around me wasn't a home anymore. It was a crime scene, and I was both the victim and the perpetrator. Emma's drawings still clung to the fridge, their corners curled and faded like they knew they'd been abandoned. Lucas's trucks sat exactly where he'd last played with them. Untouched, collecting dust. The silence in their rooms screamed louder than any fight Jake and I ever had. I used to tuck them in. Now, those rooms just stored empty wine bottles and unopened bills I couldn't face.

I hadn't seen them in twelve weeks.

Supervised visits were the only way, but those came with rules. Sobriety tests, scheduled appointments, meetings with social workers. I hadn't passed one. Not even close. I was either too drunk to show up or too ashamed to try. Jake stopped reaching out after the third time I showed up hours late and clearly intoxicated. I still remember the last time the social worker whispered to him, not realizing I could hear through the thin walls.

"She's not ready," she said. "We have to put the kids first."

They were right.

Emma had turned seven. Lucas was five and a half. I missed both birthdays. Jake sent a photo of Emma holding a cake, her front teeth missing, her eyes looking through the camera like she was searching for someone who wasn't there. I stared at it for hours. I never replied.

Jake was raising them now. He helped with homework, cheered at soccer games, brushed their hair, packed their lunches. He got to be the stable one. The safe one. The present one.

And me?

I was face down on a bathroom floor, my stomach a twisted mess of ulcers and acid, my mouth stained with red that wasn't wine this time. The blood was new, but the warning signs had been there. Shaky hands, the dull yellow creeping into my skin, the way I dry-heaved every morning before my first drink.

I drank to stop the shaking. I drank to fall asleep. I drank so I wouldn't have to feel what it meant to be a mother who couldn't be a mother anymore.

That day, I pulled myself up using the sink like a walker. The mirror didn't reflect me. It showed someone thinner, paler, older. My cheeks were hollow, my eyes sunken. I'd lost maybe twenty pounds, not by trying, but because I couldn't keep food down. My body rejected anything that wasn't alcohol.

I shuffled through the apartment like a ghost, stepping over broken glass and pizza boxes. I couldn't remember the last time I'd done laundry. My bedroom smelled like a bar after closing. Stale wine, sweat, and something darker I didn't want to name.

The eviction notice was still taped to the door, dated two weeks earlier. I'd seen it. I just couldn't do anything about it. I'd stopped paying rent when the child support ended. Jake wasn't obligated to send anything while the kids weren't with me. My unemployment checks had dried up. I was living on credit cards and the last few dollars of the savings account we once built together.

That money was gone. My children were gone. And soon, the apartment would be gone too.

The phone buzzed on the counter. Seventeen missed calls from my mom.

I didn't answer. Not because I didn't love her, but because I didn't want her to hear the slur in my voice. I didn't want her to know that her daughter (the one who graduated with honors, who used to throw dinner parties and pack school lunches) was now hiding in a dark kitchen, too drunk to pick up the phone.

I'd built my life around two little kids, and now they were growing up without me.

That afternoon on the bathroom floor, my body said what my heart had been screaming for months.

Enough.

But even then, I wasn't ready to listen.

The refrigerator held three bottles of wine and nothing else.

No food. No milk. No juice. No signs of life. Just wine. The only thing I could keep down. The only thing that silenced the creature clawing at my gut, the one that screamed every time I tried to eat or think or feel.

My hands shook so badly it took three tries to open the bottle. The cork finally gave way with a soft pop, a sound as familiar now as the voices of my children used to be. I poured the wine like always. Steady, practiced, automatic. The first sip lit a fire in my throat. The second quieted it. By the third, the pain in my stomach dulled into something I could pretend to ignore.

This was what survival had become. Wake up sick. Drink until the shaking stops. Pass out. Repeat.

No job to go to. No school lunches to pack. No crayons scattered across the floor, no tiny shoes by the door, no little arms around my neck. No children to live for. Just this body, this bottle, this day.

The laptop on the coffee table sat open like a witness. Its screen glowed with the evidence of the week I'd spent researching the unthinkable.

How many sleeping pills does it take? Peaceful ways to die. Writing goodbye letters.

I'd written those letters three times. Each time, I deleted them. Not because I didn't mean them, but because I didn't know how to say it.

How do you explain to your children that their mother, who once sang in the car and made up bedtime stories, had chosen wine over staying alive? How do you tell your parents, who saved and sacrificed to send you to college, that their successful daughter had stopped believing she was worth saving?

The pills sat on the counter, lined up beside my wine glass. I'd bought them a week ago. Just in case. They were supposed to work gently if mixed with enough alcohol. Just sleep, the websites promised. No pain. No panic. Just silence. No more nights aching with shame. No more mornings waking to a life I couldn't face. No more missing Emma's voice or Lucas's laugh.

My phone buzzed again. Another text from my mom. "Emily, please call me. I'm worried about you. Dad and I love you."

I stared at it for a long time, trying to remember what it felt like to be loved without condition. My parents had been here twice since I lost the kids. Each time they found me drunk, unrecognizable. They'd offered help. Rehab. A place to stay. Money. A way out.

But I'd been too proud. Too ashamed. Too far gone to say yes.

Now that pride felt like a luxury I couldn't afford.

I picked up the phone and tried to type. My fingers trembled, too unsteady for full sentences. I deleted and retyped. Started over. Then settled on something simple. Something that could pass for normal if they needed it to, but might still say everything I didn't have the words for:

"Love you too. Always remember that I love you and Dad more than you'll ever know. You were the best parents anyone could ask for."

I hit send before I could change my mind.

Then I poured another glass of wine and looked at the pills again.

Somewhere inside me, the smallest, quietest voice. The part of me, not soaked in alcohol, whispered that this was a permanent decision made during a temporary storm. But that voice was faint now, barely audible beneath the exhaustion.

I wasn't sad. I was tired.

Too tired to pretend anymore. Too tired to keep trying to be someone I clearly wasn't.

Jake would marry someone stable. Someone kind. Someone who'd braid Emma's hair and clap at her recitals. Someone who'd teach Lucas to ride a bike and talk to him about dinosaurs. Someone who would show up. Someone doesn't have to be me.

And they'd be okay.

They already were.

If I left now, they could grow up saying their mom died from an illness, which was true enough. Addiction was an illness. I just wasn't strong enough to treat it.

I lined up the pills carefully. Thirty. That should be enough.

I filled a glass of water and sat at the kitchen table.

I looked around the apartment one last time.

A lot of fun memories. This was where Emma learned to ride her bike in the hallway, shouting, "Look at me, Mommy!" until I cried from pride. Where Lucas took his first steps. Wobbly and determined, falling into my arms like I was the safest place on Earth. Where we made pancakes on lazy Saturdays, read Goodnight Moon a hundred times, laughed until our stomachs hurt playing pretend games only we understood. A smile tugged at my lips as memories of my children filled my mind. Soft and warm while a single tear slipped down my cheek.

This was the place where I lost everything. Now, I have nothing to lose.

And now, it would be the place where I left it all behind.

It was also where I'd chosen alcohol over my children, day after day, until the choice wasn't mine anymore.

I picked up the first pill.

My phone rang.

I almost ignored it. But the ringtone was the one I'd set for my mother. The gentle chime that used to make me smile when I still felt like someone worth calling. The timing stopped me. She'd read my message. Twenty minutes had passed. Had it sounded as much like goodbye as I'd meant it to?

"Hello?" My voice cracked, raw from vomiting and crying.

"Emily." Her voice was sharp, breathless with panic. "I got your text. Where are you?"

"I'm home," I said. "At the apartment."

"Are you okay? You sound... different."

I looked at the mess around me. The wine bottles. The pills. The eviction notices on the floor, trampled like everything else I'd let fall apart. "I'm not okay," I said. The first truly honest thing I'd said to anyone in months.

"What's wrong? Talk to me."

"Everything," I said. "I lost my job. I'm losing the apartment. I haven't seen the kids in three months. And I can't stop drinking long enough to fix any of it."

There was silence. I could hear her breathing, could picture her hand over her mouth, trying to hold herself together on the other end of the line.

"Are you drinking right now?" she asked softly.

"Yes."

"How much have you had today?"

I glanced at the empty bottles. The half-full glass in my hand. "I don't know," I said. "I don't keep track anymore."

"Okay," she said, steady now, purposeful. "Emily, I'm coming to get you. Don't go anywhere. Don't do anything. Just wait for me."

"Mom... you don't understand. I'm too far gone. There's no coming back from this."

"There is always a way back," she said fiercely. "Always. You are my daughter, and I love you. I am not giving up on you, even if you've given up on yourself."

"I've lost everything. I am done now," I whispered.

"You've lost things that can be rebuilt. Your job. Your home. Even custody. But if you give up... if you do something you can't undo, then it's really over. And I don't want to bury my daughter."

The pills were still there, lined up in front of me. But her voice was piercing through the fog. She was driving to me. She wasn't going to let me vanish.

Someone still believed I was worth saving.

"I don't know how to get better," I said, shaking.

"You don't have to know how. You just have to want to. Do you want to get better?"

Did I?

Part of me still wanted the peace of not existing. Of not feeling. But another part (a quiet, persistent flicker) sounded like Emma's voice asking if Mommy was coming home. That part wanted to try.

"I want to see my children again," I said.

"Then we'll make that happen. But first, we get you sober. Not just dry sober. Really sober. And we'll help. Your dad and I... we're coming. We're here."

"I've tried, Mom. I've tried so many times."

"This time, you're not alone."

I swept the pills into my hand and stumbled to the bathroom. I flushed them before I could second-guess the decision. It wasn't heroic. It wasn't triumphant. It was just necessary. One step to remove the option. Making it harder to disappear.

"I'm scared," I said.

"I know you are. But you've always been brave, Emily. Even when you didn't think so."

I didn't feel brave. I felt broken. Sick. Exhausted.

"How long until you get here?" I asked.

"Twenty minutes. Can you wait twenty minutes?"

I looked around the apartment. At the mess. The wreckage. The proof of everything I'd lost.

"I can wait twenty minutes," I said.

But I couldn't.

Ten minutes after I hung up, the pain in my abdomen exploded. It was like something inside me had ruptured. I collapsed on the kitchen floor, vomiting blood again. Worse this time. So much worse. My head spun, and a low roar filled my ears, like wind in a tunnel or a train I couldn't stop.

I tried to crawl to my phone.

My arms didn't work.

The room blurred at the edges.

And my last thought, as the darkness closed in, was that my mother was going to find me like this. And she'd blame herself for not driving faster.

I woke up in a hospital bed three days later.

The first thing I saw was my mother's face. Pale, drawn, and edged with the kind of exhaustion that only comes from watching your child almost die. She hovered over me, one hand near my shoulder, like if she let go, I might disappear again.

There were tubes in my arms. A monitor beeped steadily somewhere behind me. My mouth tasted like metal, like I'd been sucking on pennies.

"Thank God...," she whispered, her voice breaking as our eyes met. "Oh, thank God..."

I tried to speak, but all that came out was a dry croak. "What... happened?"

"You almost died," she said, her voice trembling but steady. "Internal bleeding from your stomach lining. The doctor said if I'd found you an hour later..."

She didn't finish. She didn't have to.

A few minutes later, a doctor I didn't recognize stepped up to my bedside. Dr. Martinez. She had kind eyes and the practiced tone of someone who'd given news like this too many times before.

"Mrs. Matthews," she said, "you're very lucky to be alive. The amount of alcohol in your system when you came in would have killed most people. And the internal bleeding nearly did."

"How bad is it?" I asked.

She didn't soften it.

"Bad enough that if you keep drinking, you'll be dead within six months. Your liver is severely damaged. Your stomach lining is eroded. Your body's been slowly shutting down from months of alcohol poisoning."

The words landed like facts, not fear. I felt strangely detached, like she was talking about someone else's body. Someone else's slow-motion suicide.

"And if I stop?" I asked.

"If you stop completely and get real medical care, there's a chance you'll recover. Not a promise. A chance. You're still young, which helps. But some damage might be permanent."

I didn't ask about my career or my apartment or the unopened bills in a box somewhere. I didn't ask about the eviction or the job I'd lost. I asked the only question that mattered.

"What about my children?"

Dr. Martinez glanced at my mother, then back at me. "Recovery takes time. And trust, especially from family court, takes even longer. You'll have to prove you've changed. Not just for a month. Not just when it's convenient. For real. Consistently. But yes, it's possible."

Emma and Lucas. Seven and five and a half now. I hadn't seen them in twelve weeks.

I thought about the last time I held them. About telling Emma everything would be perfect. About Lucas wrapping his arms around my legs and asking if Mama was sad. About Jake, and how much safer they probably were without me. About the social worker's quiet verdict: "She's not ready."

Then I thought about the woman I used to be. The one who graduated magna cum laude, who believed in hard work and family and doing the right thing. The one who swore she'd never become her worst fear. That woman felt like a ghost. But maybe she wasn't gone.

Maybe she was just buried. And maybe, just maybe, she was ready to claw her way back.

"I want to get better," I said quietly. "I want to get sober. And stay sober. And earn the right to see my children again."

Dr. Martinez didn't smile. She didn't offer comfort or platitudes.

"This will be the hardest thing you've ever done," she said.

"Good," I replied. "Because losing them was easy. I just had to keep drinking and let it all fall apart. Getting them back should be hard."

My mother squeezed my hand. She didn't speak, but her hand trembled against mine. And in that small gesture, I felt something I hadn't felt in months.

Not forgiveness. Not absolution.

Hope.

It was small, fragile, almost ridiculous. But it was there.

And it had to be enough because I'd already fallen as far as I could.

This was rock bottom: a hospital bed, nearly dead from alcohol, with nothing left but the wreckage of what used to be my life.

But even rock bottom, I realized, could be a foundation. And maybe, if I worked like hell, stayed sober, and never forgot what I'd almost lost, I could build something new on top of it.

Something that included Emma and Lucas. Something like the life I'd once promised them. Something that might even resemble the mother I used to believe I could be.

Chapter Nine

The Visit That Changed Everything

THE FAMILY SERVICE WAITING room smelled like industrial disinfectant and broken dreams. I sat on a hard plastic chair, back straight, hands folded in my lap to keep them from shaking. Across the room, a mother tried to coax her toddler into a puzzle while her older son sulked in the corner. Nobody made eye contact. Everyone was waiting for something they'd already lost, hoping they might earn it back under fluorescent lights and a clipboard's watch.

This is where you came to prove you could be trusted again. This is where they sent parents who had failed. This is where I belong now.

It had been ninety days since I woke up in a hospital bed with my mother beside me and a doctor explaining how close I'd come to dying. Ninety days since I'd poured the last bottle of wine down the sink. Ninety days since I'd seen my children.

The clock on the wall ticked closer to 2:00 PM.

"Emily Matthews?"

I looked up. A woman with a clipboard approached with a smile that was polite, not quite warm. "I'm Claire Jennings," she said. "I'll be supervising today's visit."

I stood too fast and caught myself. Everything I did now had weight. My posture, my tone, my energy. All of it would be observed, documented, and sent to a judge who would decide whether I could be alone with my own kids again.

"Thank you," I said, relieved my voice didn't betray the storm inside. "I'm ready."

She nodded. "Emma and Lucas are already in Room B with their father."

I followed her down a hallway that felt longer than it was.

"Before we go in," she said, "I need to go over a few ground rules. This is a two-hour supervised visit. I'll be present the entire time and will take notes for my report to the court."

I nodded.

"No physical discipline. No conversations about the custody case, the divorce, or your recovery. No talk of substance use at all. And if the children ask, you're to redirect the conversation. Understood?"

Each word landed like a quiet sting, a reminder of the damage I'd done. I nodded again. This was the cost, and I was willing to pay it.

"One more thing," Claire added, her voice softening. "It's been three months. Kids don't track time like we do. They may be hesitant at first. Don't take it personally if they need time to warm up."

I swallowed hard. Warm up to their mother. That's who I was now: a visitor. Someone they had to relearn how to trust.

Claire opened the door. I stepped inside.

My heart pounded as she led me toward Room B. Through the narrow glass window, I saw Jake at a tiny table, reading to Lucas. Emma sat beside them, hunched over a workbook, her blonde ponytail swaying as she colored.

They both looked older.

It had only been three months, but kids don't wait. They'd stretched and matured in the time I'd been gone, the way children do when you're not watching. Lucas's baby face had thinned out, and Emma, my God, Emma, looked like a little adult, with that serious expression she wore when she was concentrating.

Jake looked up first. There was something behind his eyes I couldn't name. Surprise, maybe. Or relief that I looked like a human being again. The last time he saw me, I'd been bloated and glassy-eyed. Now I was twenty pounds heavier, color back in my skin, light back in my eyes. Three months sober had brought back pieces of me I thought were gone for good.

"Emma, Lucas," Jake said gently, closing the book. "Mommy's here."

Emma glanced up. For a second, she just stared at me, like her brain was buffering, trying to load a memory she wasn't sure was real. I watched her face shift: confusion, recognition, then something softer. Something like hope.

"Mommy?" she asked.

"Hi, sweetheart." I didn't move toward her. I let her decide. "You look so big. Have you grown a whole foot since I saw you last?"

That got a smile. Just a little one. "Not a whole foot," she said. "Maybe just inches."

Lucas peeked over the edge of the book, his eyes wide and cautious. He stared at me, quiet and still, until he finally spoke. "Mama?"

That one word nearly undid me.

"Hi, my sweet boy." I swallowed the lump in my throat. "I missed you so much."

Jake stood and grabbed his coat. "I'll be back at four," he told Claire. Then to the kids: "Be good for Mommy, okay?"

"Daddy's leaving?" Lucas's voice turned small, and unsure.

"Just for a little while," I said quickly. "He'll be back soon. But right now, we get to hang out. Just us."

When Jake left, the silence hit hard. It was awkward and huge, the kind of silence that fills rooms where something sacred used to live.

Emma went back to coloring, but her eyes kept flicking up at me. Lucas stayed glued to his seat, clutching his book like it could shield him from whatever came next.

I pulled up one of the tiny plastic chairs beside Emma. "What are you working on?"

"A family picture," she said, holding it up. "That's Daddy, and me, and Lucas, and Grandma and Grandpa."

I looked at the drawing and noted who was in it, and who wasn't. "It's beautiful," I said. "You've gotten so good. Have you been practicing a lot?"

"Daddy signed me up for art class. I can draw horses now."

"I'd love to see one of your horses."

Lucas inched closer, curiosity softening his edges. "Mama," he said, peering into my face, "your eyes look different."

My breath caught. "Different how?"

"They're not sleepy anymore."

Five years old, and somehow, he said it perfectly. He didn't know the word sober, but he didn't need to.

"You're right," I said. "I was really tired before. But I'm feeling better now."

"Are you not sick anymore?" he asked, climbing into the chair next to mine.

"I'm getting better every day," I said, careful not to oversell it, careful to tell the truth.

"Will you come to my soccer game?" Lucas asked, like the idea had been waiting inside him for weeks. "Daddy said maybe you could come watch."

I glanced at Claire. She gave a small nod.

"I would love to," I said. "When is it?"

"Next Saturday! I'm on the Sharks. I'm not that good yet, but Daddy says I'm improving."

"I bet you're amazing," I said, and he lit up like a Christmas tree.

Emma had been listening. She set her crayon down and looked straight at me. "Mommy," she said, "why did you go away for so long?"

My stomach clenched. Claire had warned me. Don't get into it. Don't talk about recovery or alcohol or anything messy.

But kids don't ask on a schedule. They ask when their hearts need answers.

"Sometimes grown-ups have to take time to figure out how to be better," I said slowly. "I had some problems, and I needed to work on fixing them, so I could be the kind of mommy you deserve."

Emma didn't blink. "What kind of problems?"

"The kind that made me tired and sad and not very good at taking care of the people I love most."

She studied me, far too serious for a seven-year-old. "You do look different. Happier."

"I feel happier. Especially today. Being with you and Lucas makes me feel like myself again."

There was a pause. Then Emma asked, "Can you help me with my math homework? Daddy tries, but he's not as good at explaining it as you were."

I almost laughed and was afraid I'd cry instead. She was asking me to be her mom again. Not in theory. In real life.

"I'd love to help," I said. "What are you working on?"

She pulled a sheet from her backpack. "Fractions. I hate them."

"Everyone does," I said. "But you're lucky. You've got the best tutor in the world."

Emma handed me the paper. Lucas leaned his head on my shoulder. And for the first time in a long time, I felt like maybe I could do this. Maybe not all at once, and not without work, but maybe I could earn my way back to being their mom.

One soccer game. One math sheet. One visit at a time.

We spent the next hour on math problems, Emma focused and precise, Lucas chiming in with wild guesses that made all three of us laugh. I corrected him gently, grateful for his enthusiasm, his voice, his presence beside me.

For a little while, it felt almost normal. Like we were just a mom and her kids, hanging out on a Saturday afternoon. But every time I let myself relax, I'd glance over and see Claire quietly taking notes in the corner. And I'd remember exactly where we were and why.

"Can we draw now?" Emma asked, closing her workbook and pushing it aside.

"Absolutely," I said, clinging to anything that let me stay in this moment a little longer.

She handed me a blank page and a handful of crayons. "Draw yourself."

I sketched a stick figure with long hair and a smile. Simple, but clear enough that Lucas immediately said, "That's you!"

"Now you," I told Emma, passing her the blue crayon.

She picked up two instead. When she finished, she held up a picture of two stick figures side by side. One had a frown and dark circles under its eyes, drawn in rough, heavy strokes. The other was smiling brightly, with wide, clear eyes and light, bright colors.

"This is Sad Mommy," she said, pointing to the first one. "And this is Happy Mommy."

It was like being punched in the chest. Not because I didn't understand but because I did.

"Which one am I today?" I asked carefully.

Emma studied me with her expression serious and still. "Today you're Happy Mommy."

I swallowed hard. "I remember Sad Mommy too," I said. "And I'm working really hard to make sure she doesn't come back."

"Good," Emma said simply. "I like Happy Mommy better."

"So do I," I said, and meant it.

Lucas, who'd been watching silently from across the table, suddenly climbed into my lap. The warmth and weight of his little body was almost too much. I wrapped my arms around him and held on tight.

"Mama," he said quietly, "I missed you."

"I missed you too, baby," I whispered into his hair. "So much."

Emma leaned in on my other side. And for a moment (a real, solid, soul-deep moment), we were us again. Not in our old life. Not in our old home. But us. Tangled together, warm and breathing and real.

"Will you come again soon?" Emma asked.

"If I keep working hard to stay healthy, yes," I said. "Would you like that?"

Both kids nodded. "Yes."

Tears threatened, but I blinked them back. I didn't want to waste a second of what we had left.

Claire checked her watch. "Fifteen minutes," she said quietly.

The kids felt it too. Their energy shifted. Lucas clung harder. Emma scooted closer. They were trying to store it all up to make two hours last through a whole week.

"I don't want you to go," Lucas said, his voice small and fierce.

"I don't want to go either," I told him. "But I promise, this isn't the last time. We'll see each other again."

"Do you really promise?" Emma asked, her eyes suddenly sharper. "Not like before. Not like when you used to say, 'just one more sip of wine,' and then forget?"

That one landed. Not like a punch. Not even like a slap. More like a scalpel. Sharp, precise, unforgettable.

She remembered. Of course she remembered.

"I promise differently now," I said. "I promise the way Happy Mommy promises. Not like Sad Mommy did."

Emma nodded slowly, like my answer passed some kind of test.

At exactly 4:00 PM, Jake walked in. Lucas was still on my lap. Emma stood but stayed close.

Jake looked at Claire. "How did it go?"

"Very well," she said, and I let myself breathe.

"Can we see Mommy next week?" Emma asked.

Jake glanced at me, then at Claire. "We'll have to see what the court says," he said carefully.

The kids began gathering their things. Emma ran back to the table, digging into her art supplies.

"This is for you," she said, handing me a folded piece of paper.

I opened it. On the front, two stick figures holding hands. One big, one small. Both smiling. Inside, in her careful, looping handwriting, she'd written:

"Dear Mommy, I love both Mommies, but I like this one better. Love, Emma."

I smiled, told her it was perfect, that I would keep it forever. Then I excused myself to the bathroom, locked the door, and cried silently into my hands.

When I came out, Jake and the kids were waiting by the exit.

"Emily," Jake said, his voice low, "you look... good. Really good."

"I feel good," I said. "Better than I have in a long time."

He looked at me for a moment, then down at the kids. "They missed you," he said. "More than I thought they would."

"I missed them too. Every day."

Jake nodded. "Keep doing what you're doing. For them."

"I will," I said. And for the first time in years, I didn't feel like I was lying.

I stood by the window as they walked to the car. Lucas held Jake's hand. Emma skipped beside them. Just before they got in, they both turned and waved. Big, exciting waves, like I was someone they were proud to know.

They looked happy. But I could see the confusion in their eyes too.

They were trying to understand who I was now. And maybe, for the first time, I was too.

I drove home to the small studio apartment my parents were helping me afford while I pieced my life back together, feeling like I'd just been through a storm that left me cracked open.

There was joy. Real joy. I'd held my children, heard them laugh, watched them study my face like they were searching for the mom they remembered. And for the first time in a long time, I hadn't looked away.

There was hope, too. That they still loved me. That they wanted more visits. That maybe, just maybe, I hadn't lost them forever.

But beneath the joy and hope was something heavier: the weight of all I'd broken. The damage I'd done. The long road ahead. I knew how easily I could still fail. How fragile everything still was.

The old me would've pulled into a liquor store. Just to take the edge off. Just to "celebrate" or "cope" or avoid feeling the full force of it all.

But the new me (the one who was trying) drove straight home, locked the door, and picked up the phone.

I called Linda, my sponsor, and told her everything. I didn't leave out the hard parts. The sharp question from Emma. The sting of seeing Sad Mommy in a crayon drawing. The way Lucas said, "Mama," like it still belonged to me.

"How do you feel?" Linda asked when I'd finished.

I looked at Emma's card, propped up on my tiny kitchen table. Two smiling stick figures holding hands.

"Grateful," I said. "Terrified. Hopeful. Like I was just handed something precious I don't deserve but can't bear to lose."

"Good," Linda said gently. "That's exactly where you should be. Now, what are you going to do to make sure you earn the next visit?"

I stared at the drawing again. The bright eyes. The simple words. The truth in them.

"Whatever it takes," I said. "Absolutely, whatever it takes."

And for the first time since losing my children, I believed those words might actually be enough. Not because recovery had suddenly become easy but because Happy Mommy was real now. And she was worth fighting for.

So were Emma and Lucas.

And so was the promise I'd made to never go back to being the mother they used to wait for. The one who always had just one more sip before she could show up.

Starting now, I'd show up. I'd keep my promises. And I'd never be Sad Mommy again.

Chapter Ten

The New Mrs. Matthews

THE CALL CAME ON a Tuesday night while I was making dinner. Grilled cheese and tomato soup, the only meal I could cook without setting off the smoke detector. Six months sober, and I was starting to feel like a real person again. Like maybe this recovery thing wasn't just a phase or a fluke.

When my phone buzzed, I wiped my hands on a dish towel and glanced at the screen.

Jake.

He only called if it was about Emma or Lucas. We'd just finalized my supervised visit schedule the week before, so whatever this was, it wasn't logistics. And it wasn't casual. Jake didn't do casual talks with me anymore. Every conversation was structured and sterile, like he was speaking to a polite stranger, not the woman he once promised forever.

I answered. "Hey."

"Hi. It's Jake," he said, as if I wouldn't recognize his voice. There was a tightness to it, formal, almost rehearsed.

"Everything okay?" I asked, turning down the burner under the pan. "Are the kids alright?"

"They're fine. They're great, actually." He paused. "This isn't about them, not exactly. I just wanted to tell you something before the kids do."

My stomach dropped. No good conversation ever started with, "I wanted you to hear it from me."

"Okay," I said, bracing myself.

"I'm engaged," he said in a single exhale. "Rebecca and I are getting married."

I sat down carefully, like my chair was the only thing holding me to the floor.

I'd been piecing together months of clean time, building trust with my sponsor, working the steps, staying present. While I was making soup and celebrating small victories like paying my electric bill on time, Jake had been falling in love with the woman who took care of our son in the hospital.

"That's..." I swallowed hard. "That's wonderful. Congratulations."

It tasted like metal coming out of my mouth, but I said it anyway. Because it was the right thing to say. Because I wasn't allowed to fall apart just because my ex-husband had found someone new.

Someone stable. Someone who didn't blow up their marriage with wine and secrets and lies.

"Thanks," he said, and I heard the tension drop from his voice. He'd been bracing for a reaction, maybe even a meltdown. But I was six months sober. Meltdowns weren't my thing anymore.

"We haven't told the kids yet," he added. "We're planning to this weekend. I just wanted you to know before they said something."

I nodded, forgetting he couldn't see me. "How are they with her?"

"They love her," he said. "She's been around for a few months now, just as a friend at first. She didn't push it. She's been careful. Gentle with them."

Of course she had. Of course they loved her.

She was probably the kind of woman who packed organic snacks and remembered which kid liked the red spoon. The kind of woman who didn't get drunk on school nights or miss pickup because she'd passed out on the couch.

"I'm happy for you," I said. And somehow, I meant it, at least a little.

Jake deserved happiness. He'd held our family together as long as he could before it cracked under my addiction. He'd taken care of our kids when I couldn't take care of myself. He deserved love that didn't come with caveats or court supervision.

But I couldn't stop the ache blooming in my chest.

"Rebecca wants to meet you," he said. "The kids talk about you a lot. She'd like to say hello. Just... put a face to the name."

The kids talk about you. Like I was folklore. A bedtime story about the mom who used to live with them, the one who drew horses, knew how to explain math problems, and promised things she never delivered.

I pressed my palm flat against the kitchen table, grounding myself.

"Yeah," I said. "Sure. I'd like to meet her."

In that moment, I wasn't sure if I was trying to prove something to Jake, to her, or to myself. Maybe all three. Maybe none.

But I knew this: I had to keep showing up. Even if it hurts. Even if the new Mrs. Matthews tucked my kids in at night.

Because I was still their mom. And I was still here.

We met at a coffee shop the following Saturday. Neutral ground, somewhere between my broken past and their picture-perfect present. I spent the week leading up to it in quiet dread, imagining what she was like, how she'd stepped into the wreckage I'd left behind and built something safe for my kids. Something Jake could love.

When I walked in, I knew immediately: Rebecca Collins was everything I wasn't.

She stood to greet me with a soft, open smile. Petite, elegant without trying, carrying herself with the calm assurance of someone who had nothing to prove. Her long black hair was pulled into a simple ponytail that still looked stylish. Her sweater was the kind of soft blue that made people trust you, and her eyes were warm, kind, and disarming.

I was overdressed in all the wrong ways. Too much makeup trying to fake rested, a shirt that tried too hard to say, "I'm okay now."

"Emily," she said warmly, extending her hand. "It's so nice to finally meet you. I've heard a lot about you."

I wondered what she meant by a lot. Had Jake told her everything? About the affair, the blackouts, the police, the hospital?

I shook her hand. "Nice to meet you too."

She gestured to the seat across from her. "I know this must be hard," she said gently. "But I wanted to thank you."

I blinked. "Thank me?"

"Emma and Lucas are incredible kids. Smart, sweet, funny, resilient. I know that comes from you."

That cracked something in me.

Nobody had said anything like that in a long time. For so long, all I'd heard was what I'd done wrong, what I'd lost, how far I'd fallen. But here she was, giving me credit for something good. And the worst part? She meant it.

"Thank you," I said, clearing my throat before I could cry. "They really are amazing."

"Emma told me you taught her how to braid her hair," Rebecca said with a smile. "She's been teaching me the way you showed her."

That hit harder than I expected. It could have felt like erasure, like she was slowly replacing me in the small rituals that once made me Mom. But it didn't. It felt... tender. Like a piece of me was still woven into Emma's life, even when I wasn't there to see it.

We talked for almost an hour. About the kids. School, friends, bedtime routines. Lucas had recently declared himself a paleontologist. Emma was deep in an "abstract expressionism" phase, painting everything with dramatic flair. Rebecca asked thoughtful questions and really listened. She wasn't humoring me. She wanted to know them. To get it right.

That was the most brutal part: she was kind. Genuinely, disarmingly kind.

She didn't flinch when I mentioned things I'd missed. She didn't offer advice or pity. She just sat there, present and steady. The kind of woman I might have been if I hadn't imploded my life with alcohol.

"I want you to know," she said as we stood to leave, "I'm not trying to replace you. I know I never could. I wouldn't want to. You're their mother. That's sacred."

I nodded, feeling the lump in my throat. "But you'll be their stepmother."

"Yes," she said gently. "But only because you can't be there right now. I hope someday you can."

I drove home in a fog, emotionally gutted. Her kindness was harder to handle than judgment would've been. If she'd been cold or smug, I could've found a way to hate her. But she wasn't. She was lovely. And that made everything worse.

That night I called Linda and sobbed into the phone.

"She's perfect," I choked. "She's everything I wasn't. And my kids love her. And I can't even blame them."

Linda listened without rushing me. "Of course, you feel that way," she said when the crying slowed. "You're grieving. This is grief."

"I wanted to drink so badly," I whispered. "I wanted to forget the whole day."

"But you didn't."

"No," I said. "But I wanted to."

"That's the difference now," Linda said. "You want to drink, but you don't. You feel pain, and you stay. That's recovery."

It didn't feel brave. It just felt raw. But raw was better than numb. Numb had nearly killed me.

So, I kept going.

I added more meetings. I got a therapist. I volunteered at a women's shelter because I needed to be around mothers who were still fighting too.

I did everything I could to build a life worth coming home to.

Not because I wanted to outshine Rebecca.

But because Emma and Lucas still had a mother.

And she was fighting her way back. One braid. One bedtime story. One sober day at a time.

Two months later, Jake called again.

"The kids want to invite you to the wedding," he said, skipping small talk and going straight into it like ripping off a Band-Aid.

I almost dropped the phone.

"What?"

"Emma asked if you could come to see Daddy marry Miss Rebecca. She said it wouldn't be right if you weren't there."

I swallowed hard. "And what did you tell her?"

"I told her I'd ask you. Rebecca thinks it's a lovely idea, if you're comfortable with it."

Of course, Rebecca thought it was a lovely idea. Kind, perfect, always-considerate Rebecca. Gracious even when no one would expect her to be.

"When is it?" I asked.

"Six weeks from Saturday. It's small, just close friends and family. Nothing extravagant."

Six weeks. That's how long I had to prepare myself to watch the man I once married promise forever to someone else. To smile while my children played flower girl and ring bearer for a woman who now braided their hair and helped with homework.

"I'll be there," I said, because Emma had asked. Because I was trying, with every ounce of strength I had, to be the kind of mother who shows up, even when every nerve in my body screamed to run.

"You sure?" Jake asked, quieter now. "It might be... hard."

"It will be," I said honestly. "But I'll be there."

The next six weeks felt like emotional bootcamp. I had to find something to wear that balanced appropriate and invisible. I practiced how to smile in family photos without looking like I was faking it, even though I would be. I braced myself to face the people who'd known me at my worst and would now see their relief that Jake had found someone better.

And I had to prepare to sit through a wedding reception with an open bar.

"I don't have to go," I told Linda one afternoon over coffee, my voice small and shaky. "I could back out. Blame a migraine. Spend the day at an AA meeting instead."

"You could," she said. "You have every right to protect your sobriety."

"But what would Emma think?"

Linda didn't answer. She didn't have to.

"She'd think I bailed," I said. "That I'm still the mom who disappears when things get too hard."

"Is that who you are now?"

I shook my head. "No. I'm the mom who shows up. Even when it hurts. Especially when it hurts."

"Then you know what to do."

I nodded, even though every part of me wanted to vanish. I was still grieving what I'd lost. Jake, the life we were supposed to build, the future I thought was mine. But this wasn't about me anymore. This was about Emma and Lucas. About keeping a promise I'd made to them: to be the version of myself they deserved.

Even if it meant sitting at the back of a chapel, smiling through tears, and cheering for a happy ending that wasn't mine.

Even if it meant looking at Rebecca and seeing everything I couldn't be and still choosing not to drink.

Because recovery doesn't mean you stop hurting.

It means you learn how to hurt without running away.

And that's what I was doing now.

Showing up.

Staying.

Sober.

The wedding was held at a vineyard just outside the city. Neat rows of grapes, white folding chairs under a canopy of string lights, everything picture-perfect. Emma wore a pale pink dress and carried a small bouquet of white roses. Lucas walked beside her in a miniature tuxedo, looking far too grown-up for six and a half. They were eight and nearly seven now, old enough to know this day was about building a new family. A family I would always be part of in one way, but no longer at the center.

I sat in the back row in a navy blue dress. Polished but quiet, chosen to help me blend in. I watched Jake marry the woman I used to be afraid to meet. The woman who was now part of my children's daily lives. Rebecca looked beautiful in a simple white dress with no veil, no flash, just glowing. And Jake looked peaceful in a way I hadn't seen before. There was love in his eyes, but more than that, there was steadiness. Something I had once promised and failed to give.

"I promise to love and cherish you," he said to her, "and to be the husband and father our family deserves."

Our family. He meant Emma and Lucas too. He was saying out loud what I had been trying to accept quietly for months. This marriage wasn't just about two people. It was about giving my children a safe, stable home. One I couldn't give them then. One they had now.

I cried through most of the ceremony. Not the kind of crying that ruins mascara or makes you sob, but a steady leak of complicated grief. For what I'd lost. For what they'd found. For the fact that, even though it hurt, this was good for my kids.

The reception was in a renovated barn strung with fairy lights, filled with the clink of wine glasses and polite laughter. There was an open bar. I stuck with sparkling cider and told myself it was just another Saturday night. Just another test I was ready for.

"You came," Rebecca said, finding me during cocktail hour. She looked freshly married in every possible way. Glowing, a little giddy, still floating above the rest of us.

"Emma wanted me here," I said. "And I try to show up when my kids ask me to."

"That means a lot," she said. "To them and to me. I know this can't be easy."

It wasn't. Watching Jake twirl his new wife while our children clapped was one of the hardest things I've done sober. But it was necessary. Like surgery. Painful but healing. You don't walk into something like this expecting comfort. You hope to come out intact.

During the father-daughter dance, Emma ran over to me in her pink dress and shiny shoes.

"Mommy, will you dance with me?"

"Of course, sweetheart," I said, slipping off my shoes and following her to the floor.

We swayed together, my hand on her small back, her cheek against my shoulder.

"Are you sad Daddy got married?" she asked.

"A little," I told her. "But I'm also really happy that you and Lucas have someone who takes such good care of you."

"Rebecca reads us bedtime stories," she said. "And she helps with my spelling and never yells when we're loud."

She didn't say "like you used to," but she didn't have to.

"I'm glad," I said. "You deserve someone who's patient and kind."

Emma looked up at me. "Can I call her mom? Not instead of you. You're mommy. She could be mom?"

My chest ached, but I made myself take a breath. This wasn't about me. It was about her.

"If that feels right to you," I said, steadying my voice, "then yes. That's okay."

Her face lit up. "Really?"

"Really. You can love more than one person. That doesn't take anything away from the love we already have."

She hugged me tightly. "I love you, Mommy."

"I love you too, Emma. So much."

Later, when the evening was winding down and I was gathering my things, Jake met me outside near the parking lot. The sky was dark, but the barn still glowed behind him.

"Thanks for coming," he said. "It meant a lot to the kids."

"It meant a lot to me too," I said. "Hard as it was."

He looked at me for a moment. "You look good. Really good. Healthy."

"I feel good," I said. "Better than I have in years."

"The kids noticed. Emma told Rebecca you're Happy Mommy all the time now."

That made me smile. I remembered her drawing. Sad Mommy with tired eyes, Happy Mommy with bright ones.

"I'm working on staying that way," I said.

"They need Happy Mommy."

"They need stability," I said, "which they have now with you and Rebecca."

Jake nodded. "Yeah. But they also need their mother. The real version of their mother. Not the one who was drowning in wine."

As I drove home, the vineyard lights fading in the distance, I felt scraped out but not destroyed. I'd stayed sober. I'd shown up. I'd danced with my daughter and answered her impossible questions with truth and grace. I'd kept every promise I'd made to myself that morning.

And most of all, I'd seen with my own eyes that Emma and Lucas were okay. More than okay. They were growing up, safe, and surrounded by love.

Even if I wasn't the one giving them everything, they were getting what they needed.

And that had to be enough.

For now.

The apartment was still when I got home. Soft and quiet but not hollow the way it used to feel. I put on the kettle, made a cup of tea, and sat on the edge of my small couch. Photos from my supervised visits were spread across the coffee table, each one a reminder of how far I'd come. Emma's toothy grin. Lucas in his soccer uniform. Me, smiling with both of them beside me, no wine glass in sight.

Six months ago, I'd been lying in a hospital bed, my body barely holding on. Tonight, I'd walked into my ex-husband's wedding with clear eyes, a steady heart, and a firm grip on my sobriety. I'd shaken hands with the woman who would help raise my children and managed to see her for what she was. Kind, steady, good. I watched Emma and Lucas laugh and dance and belong. Not lost. Not confused. Just okay.

I had shown up. Not perfectly. Not without pain. But fully. For them. For myself. For the woman I was still trying to become.

This wasn't the life I imagined when I first became a mother. But it was a life I could stand now without shame. A life built on truth instead of lies. On being here instead of checked out. On love that wasn't tangled up in addiction.

A life where maybe, if I kept doing the work, Happy Mommy would be more than just a visitor. She might actually get to stay.

And that was worth everything. Worth every hard morning and every sober night. Worth becoming the mother Emma and Lucas deserved, even if the path to get there was longer, harder, and lonelier than I'd ever planned.

Because recovery isn't about reclaiming the past. It's about earning the future.

Chapter Eleven

Fighting for My Place

I HAD A JOB again. Marketing coordinator at a nonprofit that supported families affected by addiction. The kind of place that actually understood what rock bottom looked like. The kind of place where my past didn't disqualify me, it qualified me.

During the interview, my supervisor, Michael, had looked me straight in the eye and said, "You get it. That's more important than any resume."

And he was right. I did get it.

My apartment was still modest with one room, fold-up bed, but it had warmth now. Books on the shelf. A calendar on the fridge with school events circled in red. A small bin of art supplies tucked in the corner for Emma. A basket of dinosaur figurines for Lucas.

Because they came over now. Not just under watchful supervision, but freely. Every other weekend and one school night a week, they came home to me. We cooked together, worked through math problems, and went to the museum. Pancakes on Saturday mornings had become a ritual. They were getting used to the rhythm of this new life, and so was I.

Emma, almost nine now. She noticed things but didn't always say them out loud. She let me relearn how to parent without making me feel like I was constantly failing. Lucas, seven and a half, still clung to the belief that Mommy had just been gone for a little while, not broken. He accepted things as they were.

It wasn't perfect. But it was ours.

When Michael stood up at the end of our team dinner and announced my promotion, it took me a second to realize he was actually saying my name.

"Emily," he said, lifting his champagne glass. "Our new Marketing Director. The board was unanimous. No one deserves this more."

The room broke into applause, and for a moment I just sat there, stunned. My cheeks flushed. Not from wine, but from something quieter and stronger: pride, real pride. The kind that stays with you after the party ends.

Eighteen months ago, I wouldn't have made it past the appetizer without downing my first glass of wine and eyeing the next. Tonight, the champagne glittered across the table like liquid gold, but the glass in front of me held sparkling cider. In this light, it looked the same. But I knew the difference. And I knew why it mattered.

I raised my glass and smiled at the people clapping for me. Not out of politeness, but because they'd seen me show up every single day, rebuild from the ground up, and never once ask for shortcuts or sympathy.

"Speech!" Janet from accounting called out, and I felt every pair of eyes swing my way.

A year and a half ago, I would've needed a drink just to breathe through this. To quiet the voice that said I wasn't enough. Tonight, I stood without hesitation. No trembling hands. No foggy mind. Just a clear, steady voice and a heart that knew exactly what this moment meant.

"Thank you," I said, scanning the room. Some of these people had no idea what I'd come back from. Others did. "When I started here, I didn't know if I'd ever be trusted with real responsibility again. This means more than I can explain."

As I spoke, I saw the bartender pop another cork at the back of the room. That familiar sound (sharp and celebratory) echoed like muscle memory. For a split second, I remembered the taste of champagne. That first cold sip. The fizzy promise of escape.

But the moment passed. Just a flicker. Nothing more.

"To second chances," I said, holding up my glass, "and to the people who believe in them."

Later, as we were grabbing coats and saying goodbyes, David from communications, not that David, pulled me aside.

"I hope this isn't too personal," he said, lowering his voice, "but I noticed you weren't drinking. Are you okay? I mean... you're not sick or anything?"

Not too long ago, a question like that would have made me feel cornered. Embarrassed. Tonight, I didn't flinch.

"I don't drink anymore," I told him. "Just a personal choice. But thanks for checking."

David looked unsure. "I hope we didn't make you uncomfortable. With all the champagne and stuff."

"Not at all," I said, and the truth of that surprised even me. "I'm exactly where I want to be. Drinking exactly what I want."

I drove home on my own without calculating how many drinks I could get away with, without mouthwash in my purse, and without shame pressing down on me. I thought about how different it all felt now. Celebration wasn't a trigger anymore. It didn't need to be followed by a drink to feel real. It was real because I'd earned it. Because I'd shown up for it. Because it wasn't an escape. It was proof I didn't need one.

Back at my apartment, I called Jake's house. He put Emma and Lucas on speakerphone, and I got to share the news the only way that mattered.

"Mommy got a promotion!" I said, and their squeals nearly broke the phone.

"Does that mean we get ice cream?" Lucas asked, which made me laugh.

"It means Mommy might be able to get a place with more room when you come stay," I said, and heard Emma gasp like I'd just promised her Disneyland.

After I hung up, I made a cup of tea and sat on the couch, staring at the framed photo of them on the coffee table. My babies. My reason.

Eighteen months sober. And I wasn't clawing back the old life anymore. I was building a new one. Honest. Steady. Quietly beautiful in all the ways I used to miss while chasing numbness.

Which is why Jake's call the following Wednesday hit me like a punch to the chest.

Everything I'd built. Everything I thought was finally solid started to shake again.

"Emily, I need to talk to you," Jake said, voice calm but stiff. That tone. The one he used when something was coming, and it wasn't going to be easy.

"Okay..." I said slowly. "What's going on?"

"I think it's better discussed in person. Can you come by Sunday? After you drop the kids off?"

His voice wasn't cold, but it was formal. Controlled. And that told me everything I needed to know. This wasn't small. This was a conversation that would matter.

"Yeah," I said. "I can come by."

I hung up the phone and just sat there in the quiet, the tea on my table growing cold.

After everything I'd worked to rebuild, the life I was finally starting to believe in, something was about to shift again. And I wasn't sure which way it would go.

Three days later, I sat on Jake and Rebecca's living room couch, the one that matched the elegant color scheme of the entire house, where everything looked curated and calm, like a photo shoot pretending to be a home. The kids were in the next room, immersed in a video game, laughing like it was just another weekend. They had no idea what was about to happen.

"Rebecca got a job offer," Jake said, skipping the small talk.

I looked at him. Then at her. She was sitting very still beside him, spine straight, hands folded tightly in her lap. Her face was calm but not relaxed.

"It's a position at Children's Hospital of Colorado," Jake continued. "Head of pediatric nursing. It's... kind of a dream role."

I turned to Rebecca again. She gave me a polite, nervous smile.

"Congratulations," I said. The word came out flat, heavy. "That's... big."

"Thank you," she said softly. "It really is. But it means... we'd have to move."

There it was. Relocate. A word that meant goodbye.

"All of you?" I asked, even though I already knew.

Jake didn't flinch. "The kids will come with us," he said. "We can't just leave them behind."

"Their mother is here too," I said. My voice was calm. Too calm.

Rebecca shifted slightly. "We've talked about ways to keep your relationship with them strong. We could plan for long visits, summers, holidays, and regular video calls..."

"Video calls," I repeated, staring at her like she'd just suggested mailing me sketches of their faces. "You want to take my children halfway across the country and offer me FaceTime as a substitute?"

"Emily," Jake said, trying for diplomacy, "this is a once-in-a-lifetime opportunity for Rebecca."

"And what about my once-in-a-lifetime? What about the relationship I've been rebuilding with my kids? The one I almost lost because of my addiction, the one I've fought for every single day for the past eighteen months?"

They didn't respond. They didn't need to. The way they looked at each other said everything. They'd already made up their minds. This conversation was just a courtesy.

"We're not trying to hurt you," Rebecca said gently. "But we also have to think long-term. This position comes with a big salary increase, great benefits, and real room to grow. It would mean a more secure future for everyone."

"Everyone but me," I said.

"That's not true," Jake said quickly. "We're not shutting you out."

"You're moving my kids across the country."

Jake took a deep breath. "We've been the ones there every day, Emily. For the school pickups and the fevers and the spelling tests. That consistency matters. We've become their foundation."

We've become their foundation. Not you're still their mother. Not you've worked hard and changed. Just we've replaced you.

It knocked the wind out of me.

"You don't get to say that," I said quietly. "You don't get to erase everything I've done because I fell apart and had to build myself back up slower than your timeline allowed."

Jake sighed. "This isn't about erasing you."

"Really?" I stood up. "Because from where I'm sitting, it sure feels like you've drawn a neat little life without me in it."

"We're trying to do what's best for the children," Rebecca said.

"The best for your family," I snapped. "You're asking me to step aside, so you can take my place without the inconvenience of me still living nearby."

"That's not fair," she started.

"Fair?" I said, my voice was rising for the first time. "I made terrible choices. I know that. I lost so much because of them. But I didn't walk away. I stayed. I got sober. I showed up. And I've been earning back every ounce of trust with my children one painful, beautiful moment at a time. And now, when we've finally found a rhythm, when they're finally letting me back in, you want to take them away?"

Jake stood now too. "It's not that simple."

"No," I said, meeting his eyes. "It is. You're choosing her job over my relationship with our children."

"I hoped it wouldn't come to this," he said quietly.

"You hoped I'd just accept it," I said. "I won't. I need to talk to a lawyer."

There was a beat of silence. Not shock, just resignation. They knew I'd say it eventually.

Rebecca looked down. Jake nodded.

I left before I said anything I couldn't take back. But as I pulled the door closed behind me, I felt it. The fight wasn't over. Not by a long shot.

Because this time, I wasn't fighting to keep a secret or to preserve an illusion. I was fighting for something real. I was fighting for my place.

Emma appeared in the doorway, her small frame tense, her eyes scanning the room like she was bracing for impact.

"Why is everyone yelling?" she asked.

Just like that, the room snapped into silence. The three of us, me, Jake, and Rebecca, stood frozen in the wreckage of our adult conversation, caught letting the storm spill into the wrong room.

"We're not yelling, sweetheart," Rebecca said quickly, her voice warm and gentle, the way she probably used when Emma scraped a knee. "We're just having a grown-up discussion."

Emma didn't buy it. She looked at each of us like she was trying to solve a puzzle with missing pieces. "Are you mad at each other?"

"No one's mad," I said, forcing a breath into my lungs. My voice came out softer this time. Controlled. "We're just talking about some changes that might happen."

She stepped into the room now, cautious. "What kind of changes?"

Jake and Rebecca looked at me, one of those unspoken passes adults make when something needs saying and no one wants to be the one to say it. I nodded.

"Daddy and Mom Rebecca might be moving to a new city," I said, choosing my words carefully, using the name Emma had settled on for her stepmother. "Because of a job she was offered."

Emma's eyes widened. "What about me and Lucas?"

"You'd go with them," I said. My voice stayed steady, but I could feel the ache building in my chest. "You'd have a new house, maybe a new school. It would be a big change."

She blinked. I could see her trying to process it all, curiosity, fear, confusion, flashing across her face in waves.

"What about you?" she asked.

I smiled softly, though it nearly broke my face to do it. "I'd stay here. But we'd still have our visits. We'd still talk. We'd make it work."

Emma turned to Jake and Rebecca, her voice climbing. "How often would we see Mommy?"

Jake hesitated, and in that pause, I realized we hadn't discussed anything beyond logistics and dreams. Not the actual children. Not what it would mean to them.

"We haven't figured that part out yet," Jake admitted.

"I don't want to move away from Mommy," Emma said, and the words hit me like a battering ram, grief and gratitude crashing into each other in my chest.

Rebecca stepped in, her voice soothing. "It would be an adventure, Em. New places to explore, different activities, maybe even a bigger room."

"But I just got used to having two houses," Emma said, her tone suddenly all logic and certainty, like only a nine-year-old could be. "And what about school? What about my friends? My art teacher?"

Behind her, Lucas had wandered into the room, rubbing his eyes like he'd just woken from a nap but knew something was off.

"Are we moving?" he asked.

"Maybe," Jake said. "Would that be exciting?"

Lucas shrugged, uncertain. "I guess. But what about Mommy's house? What about our pancakes on Saturdays?"

That was it.

I excused myself to the bathroom and cried with the door locked, pressing a hand over my mouth so they wouldn't hear the sound.

When I finally came out, eyes red and throat raw, Jake and Rebecca were sitting with the kids, their voices low and careful, explaining that nothing was set in stone. That this was just a conversation. That there would be time. That it might even be fun.

I didn't trust myself to speak much.

"I need to go," I said, reaching for my coat. "Emma, Lucas, I'll see you this weekend, okay?"

Emma stood and walked over to me with eyes still shadowed with worry. "Promise?"

"Promise," I said. I kissed both their foreheads and held them just a second longer than usual, like I could imprint the feel of them into my bones.

And then I left before I cried again. Because I didn't know how many more goodbyes like that I'd get.

Monday morning, I was back in Jennifer Walsh's office, the same attorney who'd sat across from me during the worst chapter of my life. Her desk hadn't changed, still stacked with neat piles of legal folders, still smelling faintly of coffee and printer ink. But I had.

I wasn't the trembling woman begging not to lose her kids. Not anymore.

After I explained the situation, Jennifer leaned back in her chair, hands folded thoughtfully. "They can petition for relocation," she said. "And since Jake has primary custody and has been providing day-to-day consistency, the court may side with him."

"What about me?" I asked. "What about my rights as their mother?"

"You have rights, Emily. But in family court, the gold standard is 'the best interest of the child.' If Jake and Rebecca can show that Denver offers a better environment (stronger schools, safer neighborhoods, more financial stability), the judge could approve the move."

"Even if it basically cuts me out of their lives?"

"They won't frame it that way," Jennifer said. "The court will expect you to maintain your relationship through summer visits, holidays, FaceTime, phone calls. There are parents who make long-distance custody work."

"Yeah, well, most of those parents didn't lose custody for being blackout drunk and disappearing for days at a time," I said, my voice sharp with guilt and frustration.

Jennifer didn't flinch. "That history complicates things. Your recovery is admirable, but in legal terms, it's still early. Eighteen months is a strong start, but the court may see this as a chance to offer Emma and Lucas a fresh start, one that doesn't carry the weight of your past."

"So, I'm being punished because recovery takes time," I said, the words landing hard in the quiet office.

"You're being evaluated based on who you are today," she said gently. "Not who you're becoming, or who you hope to be in five years. It's not fair, but it's how these cases are decided."

I walked out of her office hollowed out. I'd spent a year and a half clawing my way back from rock bottom, getting sober, rebuilding trust, showing up, and now all of it could be undone by someone else's job offer. One decision, and the fragile, beautiful relationship I'd been stitching back together with Emma and Lucas could unravel.

That night, I called Linda. When she picked up, I didn't bother with pleasantries.

"They're trying to take my kids to Denver," I said. "And I think they might win."

She listened silently until I stopped rambling. Then came the question she always started with.

"How are you feeling?"

"Like I want to walk into the nearest liquor store and drink everything in it," I said honestly.

"But you're not going to do that."

"No. But the thought is loud. Louder than it's been in a long time. I feel like everything I've worked for is slipping through my fingers and there's nothing I can do to stop it."

"Is that really true?" she asked. "That there's nothing you can do?"

"I can't compete with a dream job at a top hospital. I don't have a backyard or a second income. I can't offer them a bigger house or private school or ski trips."

Linda waited, letting the silence stretch until the real answer surfaced.

"What can you offer them?"

I closed my eyes and saw Emma's smile when I picked her up for our weekend visits. I thought of Lucas giggling during pancake breakfasts, the way they curled up under my arm during movie nights, the tiny drawings taped all over my fridge. I thought of the quiet, steady love that had been growing between us again. Careful, but real.

"I can offer them me," I said finally. "Not the broken version. Not the drunk. The real me. The one who's sober and shows up and keeps her promises. The one who loves them more than anything."

"Is that worth fighting for?"

"Yes," I said, and my voice didn't shake. "It is."

The custody modification hearing was scheduled for three weeks out. Three weeks to prepare for the most important fight of my life.

I spent every one of those days gathering proof. Not just of my sobriety, but of my consistency, my growth, my presence. Michael, my supervisor at the nonprofit, wrote a letter vouching for my reliability and compassion. My therapist submitted a report outlining my mental health progress. The school counselor offered to testify about how much more grounded Emma and Lucas had seemed since I'd reentered their lives.

And Linda, God bless Linda, agreed to testify as my sponsor. Not just to say I was attending meetings, but to speak about who I'd become in recovery. The way I showed up, not just for my kids, but for myself.

"The court needs to understand," I told Jennifer as we went over the prep, "that this isn't about geography. If they move to Denver, I will lose them. Not in theory. In reality. Summer visits and phone calls won't rebuild the trust I spent a year and a half earning."

Jennifer nodded. "I know. But we have to be clear-eyed about what the judge will prioritize. And be ready if the decision doesn't go your way."

We returned to the same courtroom where, two years earlier, I'd lost custody. That time, I was hungover, terrified, full of excuses.

This time, I was sober, prepared, clear. I wasn't there to beg. I was there to fight.

Jake and Rebecca's attorney went first. She spoke in polished, rehearsed tones about Denver's schools and crime statistics, about Rebecca's job title and salary, and about opportunity.

Rebecca took the stand, gracious and composed in her soft gray suit.

"Mrs. Collins," the judge said, "this is clearly an excellent professional opportunity. But explain to me why relocating is in the children's best interest, not just yours."

"I love Emma and Lucas like they're my own," she said. "This role would give us financial security and environment to provide them the best possible future."

"And their biological mother?" the judge asked. "How do you factor that relationship into the equation?"

"We've always encouraged Emily's involvement," Rebecca said carefully. "And we'd continue to involve her through holidays, summers, video calls..."

I stopped listening after that. Because no matter how kind her voice was, the reality remained: they were offering me scraps.

When it was my turn, I stood at the same witness stand where I'd once broken down, pleading with the court not to take my babies. This time, I didn't cry. I didn't plead. I just told the truth.

Jennifer asked me, "Can you describe your current relationship with Emma and Lucas?"

"I've been sober for eighteen months," I said. "That doesn't just mean I haven't had a drink. It means I've rebuilt my life, one painful piece at a time, to be someone my kids can rely on. I've shown up for them every week at pickup, at bedtime, at parent-teacher meetings, through art projects and math homework and movie nights."

"What would happen to that relationship if they moved to Denver?"

I looked at the judge, then at the empty seats where my children should've been. "It would fall apart. Not because I don't love them. But because rebuilding trust takes presence, not just promises. You don't fix the past over FaceTime."

"And what would you say to the argument that Mr. Matthews and Mrs. Collins can offer them more materially or academically?"

I swallowed hard. "What I can offer them is this: a mother who climbed her way back from the bottom of a bottle to stand here today. A mother who owns her mistakes, who fought to change, and who will never stop fighting to be in her children's lives. Yes, better schools and bigger houses matter. But so does knowing that your mother didn't give up. So does seeing her keep her promises."

Jake's lawyer came at me hard. My drinking. The custody loss. The affair. She wanted me to crack, to fall apart under pressure.

But I didn't.

"If I wanted convenience," I said quietly, "I'd let them go. But recovery taught me that convenience is a trap. What matters is doing the hard thing. The right thing. And this, fighting for them, is the right thing."

The judge spoke with Emma and Lucas in chambers. It only took twenty minutes, but they were the longest twenty minutes of my life.

Two hours later, she delivered her decision.

"This court acknowledges the benefits of relocation," she said, and my stomach twisted.

"But the court also acknowledges that Mrs. Matthews has demonstrated significant and sustained progress in her recovery. Her involvement is not just beneficial. It is foundational to the children's emotional well-being."

I held my breath.

"Mr. Matthews and Mrs. Collins are free to relocate to Denver. But the children will remain in this jurisdiction. Custody will be modified to reflect Mrs. Matthews' continued stability, with expanded visitation pending six more months of demonstrated progress."

I almost didn't hear the rest. All I could hear was the word that mattered: stay.

They were staying.

Jake sat frozen. Rebecca's jaw tightened, but she didn't protest. Their lawyer muttered about options and appeals, but I didn't care. I'd won the only thing that mattered.

Later, as Jennifer and I walked out of the building, I asked her quietly, "What did the kids say?"

She smiled. "That they love their stepmother and they're proud of their father. But they want to stay close to their mother. Emma told the judge, 'She's finally Happy Mommy all the time. We don't want to lose her again.'"

And neither, I realized, did I.

Six months later, I was spending Saturday afternoons at the children's hospital, sitting cross-legged on the floor with a stack of picture books and reading to kids recovering from surgery or treatment. It was part of my service work, something AA encouraged as a way to give back, but more than that, it grounded me. Being of use. Showing up.

That's where I met Mark Rodriguez.

He was a high school counselor who volunteered on weekends, bringing therapy dogs to sit with the kids during their recovery. We'd cross paths in the pediatric wing, him walking a golden retriever named Daisy, me reading The Gruffalo for the hundredth time.

"You're good with them," he said one afternoon, nodding toward a six-year-old girl who had just asked me to read the story again.

"I've had some practice," I said, collecting the scattered books. "I've got two of my own. Emma's ten now. Lucas just turned eight."

"They're lucky to have you."

I laughed. This time not with bitterness, but with humility. "It took me a long time to become someone they could be lucky to have."

He didn't push. Didn't ask for the backstory. Just smiled in a way that said he'd been through some things too.

Over time, we started talking more about his work with teens, my job at the nonprofit, how both of us had a front-row seat to people trying to hold their families together. We had different histories, but we shared the same belief: that second chances matter, and that the people who work for them deserve support.

Three months later, he asked me out for coffee.

We were walking to his car after our first real date when I stopped him.

"I should probably say this now," I said. "I'm a recovering alcoholic. I've got trust issues. And a complicated custody history."

He smiled. "I should probably say I'm a divorced high school counselor who's seen every shade of family dysfunction. I also believe people can change if they want it badly enough."

I looked at him and, for the first time in a very long time, I didn't feel like damaged goods.

"That might actually work," I said.

"I think so too."

I waited four months before introducing him to Emma and Lucas. Not because I didn't trust him, but because I finally trusted myself not to rush, not to confuse my hope with their readiness.

I talked it through with Jake and Rebecca first, and to my surprise, they supported the idea.

"You fought hard to keep them here," Jake said one day over coffee. We started meeting once a month to talk about the kids. "I didn't think you had that kind of fight in you."

"I didn't think I did either," I said. "But recovery shows you what you're made of. And it doesn't let you off the hook just because something is hard."

"Rebecca was disappointed about Denver," he admitted.

"I'm sorry," I said and I meant it. "It was a good opportunity."

"She ended up getting promoted here instead. Head of pediatric nursing. Not as flashy as Colorado, but she's happy."

"I'm glad. She's good for you. And good for them."

He paused. "So is sobriety," he said. "So is the mom you've become."

I let that sink in.

When I finally brought Mark into the kids' world, it was at a bowling alley. Something light. No big talk. No pressure. Just lanes and bumpers and pizza and letting everyone feel it out.

"He's nice," Emma whispered to me between turns, while Mark helped Lucas adjust his stance. "He listens when Lucas talks about space. And he didn't try to help me with bowling until I asked. Daddy used to just grab the ball and show me."

I smiled. "How would you feel if Mark and I kept spending time together?"

Emma gave me her serious ten-year-old look. "As long as you don't become Sad Mommy again, I think it's okay."

"I'm not going to be Sad Mommy again," I said. "I promise."

"Good," she said. "Happy Mommy is better."

That night, after dropping the kids off at Jake and Rebecca's, Mark and I sat on my couch, sharing a quiet moment.

"They're amazing," he said. "You've done a good job with them."

"I'm proud of them," I said. "And now, finally, I'm starting to feel like I deserve to be."

He looked at me, warm and steady. "I love that about you."

"What?"

"That you know love isn't a right. It's something you earn. And you're not afraid to earn it, over and over."

Two years sober, and I was learning what that kind of love looked like. Love that doesn't chase or cling or demand. Love that sits beside you on the hard days. That lets your kids take the lead. That makes space for mistakes and still shows up.

It wasn't the life I once imagined. It was better.

Because this life, I built sober, one right choice at a time.

And for the first time since I became a mother, I could look in the mirror and say it without flinching:

I am proud of the mother I'm becoming.

Chapter Twelve

Full Circle

Three years sober, and I found myself parked outside the place where everything had fallen apart.

The old apartment building on Maple Street. Third floor. Unit 3B. I hadn't been back since the day police officers knocked on my door, walked into my alcohol-soaked disaster of a life, and set in motion the chain of events that took my children from me.

The building looked smaller now, less threatening somehow. The paint was peeling, the lot full of potholes. A few window blinds hung crooked, and the landscaping had long since given up. It didn't scare me anymore. It just looked... tired. Like a place that had seen too much.

I didn't really know why I'd come. It was a Wednesday morning. I'd dropped Emma and Lucas off at school, my normal routine since I'd earned back overnight visits six months ago, and instead of heading to work, I'd driven here almost on autopilot.

I sat in the car for a while. Then I got out.

I stood for a long time just staring at that third-floor window. That was the place where I nearly drank myself to death. Where I lost custody. Where I looked in the mirror and didn't recognize the woman staring back. The place where "Sad Mommy" lived.

"Excuse me," a voice said behind me. "Are you okay?"

I turned to see a young woman with a toddler on her hip. She looked about twenty-five, maybe younger. Her ponytail was loose, her sweatshirt stained with something that looked like applesauce, and her eyes... God, her eyes. I knew that look. The barely-holding-it-together look. The smile that doesn't quite reach the face.

"I'm fine," I said. "Just... remembering. I used to live here. Third floor."

"Oh," she said. "We're in 3A. I'm Jessica."

"Emily," I said, offering my hand. "You live next door to where I hit rock bottom."

Jessica let out a breath that sounded like relief or exhaustion, maybe both.

"You okay?" I asked. Not just to be polite, but because I already knew the answer.

She tried to smile. "It's just... hard. Being home all day with him. No help, no break. My husband works long shifts, and when he's home, he acts like I should be grateful. Like this is easy."

I nodded, heart aching. "It's not easy. It's lonely and exhausting and invisible, and you start wondering if you're just... bad at it."

Her eyes filled. She blinked fast.

"I used to think I was the only one," I said softly. "I thought everyone else had figured it out and I was the mess. But that's the lie motherhood tells you when you're drowning."

She adjusted the toddler on her hip. Tyler, I'd later learn, and looked away like she was ashamed of saying too much to a stranger.

I opened my purse and pulled out a small stack of business cards. Not for my day job, the marketing work I did for nonprofit, but for something closer to the heart. A support group I'd started with a few other moms in recovery.

"This is for you," I said, handing her the card. "Thursday nights at the community center. It's a group for moms who are overwhelmed, exhausted, questioning everything. No pressure. Just support."

She looked down at the card, then asked, "Is it... is it for moms like me?"

"It's for moms who are trying their best," I said. "Some of us have dealt with postpartum depression. Some with anxiety. Some of us, like me, with addiction. But we've all felt like we're failing. You won't be the only one."

"Are you a therapist or something?"

I smiled. "No. I'm a marketing director. And a mom who nearly lost everything because I didn't know how to ask for help. I'm not an expert, but I am someone who's been there."

Tyler began to fuss. She bounced him gently, but her eyes stayed on the card in her hand.

"Thursday nights?" she said.

"Seven to eight-thirty. Childcare's provided. You can come just to listen. Or cry. Or sit in the back and say nothing."

Jessica nodded slowly, like she was giving herself permission to want something more.

"You're not alone," I said gently. "Even when it feels like it."

And standing there in that worn-out parking lot, outside the apartment where my world once shattered, I realized something: I hadn't come here to revisit my past. I'd come to meet someone who reminded me of it, and to show her that there's a way through.

That maybe the worst place you've ever been is the very ground where something better can start.

Driving to work after meeting Jessica, I kept thinking about how strange life is. Three years ago, I was the one standing in that parking lot. Exhausted, ashamed, and barely holding it together. Now I was the one offering someone else a way forward.

It felt surreal, like I'd somehow crossed over to the other side of a line I didn't even know existed.

As I pulled into the office parking lot, my phone rang. It was Linda.

"Hey," I answered. "Everything okay?"

"I have a situation," she said, her voice tight. "New sponsee. Mother of two. Just relapsed after eight months sober. She called me at two this morning from a hotel room with a bottle of pills and a bottle of vodka."

My stomach dropped.

"Is she okay?"

"Physically, yes. I stayed on the phone with her, talked her through it. She flushed the pills, poured out the vodka. But she's barely hanging on. Her ex just filed for full custody, and she's spiraling."

"What can I do?"

"I think she needs to hear from someone who's made it to the other side of this. Someone who lost custody, relapsed, and came back. Someone like you."

"Absolutely," I said. "When and where?"

"St. Mark's, this afternoon. Her name's Amanda. And Emily... she reminds me of you, back in the beginning."

That afternoon, I sat across from Amanda in a quiet side room at the church, and it felt like looking into a time-warped mirror. Shaky hands and her eyes hollowed out with shame and exhaustion. The kind of tired that no amount of sleep could touch.

"Linda says you lost your kids too," she said, eyes fixed on the floor.

"I did," I said. "Almost a full year. I couldn't see them without a social worker in the room."

Amanda's voice cracked. "How do you live with that? Knowing you chose drinking over your kids?"

"I didn't live with it. Not at first. It nearly destroyed me. But eventually, I realized something: guilt that just sits there turns into self-hate. But guilt that pushes you to change? That's fuel. You can use it."

Her hands were trembling in her lap. "But what if it's too late? What if they're better off without me?"

I took out my phone and pulled up a picture from last weekend. Emma and Lucas were in my kitchen, covered in flour, flipping pancakes while Mark stood behind them with a goofy grin.

"This was Saturday morning," I said, handing her the phone. "We made pancakes, went to the museum, and had a movie night. They asked me to come. It wasn't a court-mandated visit. It was their choice."

Amanda stared at the photo for a long time, blinking back tears. "How long did it take to get there?"

"Three years. Two before I had overnight visits. And even then, I had to show up every day on time, sober, stable. I had to prove over and over that I was serious. That I was trustworthy."

"I don't know if I'm that strong," she whispered.

"You don't have to be strong forever," I said. "Just today. Then tomorrow, you do it again."

We talked for two hours. About the difference between being dry and being truly sober. About showing up even when you feel like hiding. About how rebuilding trust with your kids is a slow process measured in pancakes and bedtime stories, not grand gestures.

Before Amanda left, she had a printed meeting schedule in her hand. Linda had agreed to sponsor her. And she had something else she didn't have when she walked in.

Hope.

"Thank you," she said, hugging me. "For not sugarcoating it. And for showing me it's still possible."

"It's more than possible," I told her. "If you want it badly enough, and you're willing to do the work? You can have a life so good you won't recognize it as yours."

That evening, I spoke at a women's AA meeting in the basement of the old Methodist church downtown, the one with the flickering lights and the smell of burned coffee that never quite goes away. I've been coming here for years, but now I showed up to give, not just to receive. Twice a month, I shared my story with the newcomers, women sitting in those folding chairs just like I once had, terrified and brittle and wondering if change was even possible.

"My name is Emily, and I'm an alcoholic," I began, scanning the circle of tired eyes and guarded faces. "Three and a half years ago, I nearly drank myself to death. I was alone in my apartment, drowning in vodka and shame, while my kids lived with their father because I wasn't safe to care for them."

I told them everything. About the affair, the broken marriage, the lies I'd built like scaffolding around a life that was falling apart.

About the wine bottles hidden behind books, the panic of waking up not knowing how the night ended, the suicide attempt that finally forced the truth into the open.

And then I told them about the turning point.

"I woke up in a hospital bed with a social worker on one side and my mother on the other. And in that moment, I realized I had two choices: keep drinking until it killed me or fight like hell for something better. I chose to fight."

I talked about the meetings, the steps, the long days and longer nights. I talked about learning how to be a mother again, how to sit with discomfort instead of numbing it, how to rebuild trust one small promise at a time.

"Recovery gave me back my children," I said. "But even more than that, it gave me back myself. The version of me who didn't need wine to get through a Tuesday night. The one who shows up, keeps showing up, and knows what it means to love without fear or control."

After the meeting, three women came up to me, each holding their own quiet desperation like a cracked mug they were trying not to drop.

One was a high school teacher who confessed she'd been drinking wine every night since the pandemic and couldn't stop.

One was a grandmother who'd started drinking again after her husband died and hadn't told anyone.

The third was a young mother, her voice shaking as she spoke. She reminded me so much of Jessica from that morning that it made my heart twist.

"Will you sponsor me?" she asked, eyes wide and hopeful and scared.

"I already have two sponsees," I said gently, "but I know someone who's perfect for you. Her name is Linda. She saved my life."

I gave her Linda's number and a hug, holding on a little longer than necessary because I remembered how it felt to be that raw, that desperate for connection.

As I walked to my car under the glow of the streetlamp, I realized something: this was what recovery really looked like. Not just surviving but reaching back to help the next person across the river.

And there was no part of me that missed the woman I used to be. Not even a little.

The following Saturday was Emma's eleventh birthday party, held under the wooden pavilion at Riverside Park. The sky was clear, the breeze gentle, and the air smelled like grilled hot dogs and sunscreen. Both sides of her extended family had shown up. My parents chatting easily with Jake's, the way only grandparents can when the love for a child outweighs the history between adults.

Jake and Rebecca were by the grill, flipping burgers like a well-rehearsed team. A year ago, I might've resented their ease, but not anymore. Now I saw it for what it was. Two people doing their best for the kids we all loved.

Mark was tossing a frisbee with Lucas and a group of kids from school, his laugh carrying across the field. He fit into our lives like he'd always been there, not because he forced his way in, but because he listened, stayed patient, and showed up.

"Mom," Emma said, bounding over to me with frosting smudged across her nose, "can you help me cut the cake? I want to make sure everyone gets some."

"Of course," I said, grabbing the plastic knife and following her to the table.

We stood side by side, handing out slices of chocolate cake to cousins, grandparents, school friends, and neighbors. Somewhere in the middle of frosting-covered napkins and paper plates, it hit me. This felt normal. Not forced, not staged. Just... good. Warm. Real.

Last year, something like this would've felt impossible. We were still healing, still piecing our lives back together. Now, here we were. Four adults co-parenting without drama, a blended family laughing in the park, a little girl beaming on her birthday with all her people around her.

"Emily," my mom said, coming over with a smile, "you look so happy."

"I am happy," I said. And I meant every word.

"Even after everything you've been through?"

I looked around at Lucas chasing bubbles, at Jake talking baseball with Mark, at Rebecca comforting a kid who'd scraped his knee, at Emma licking frosting off her fingers.

"Especially because of everything I've been through," I said quietly. "Losing everything forced me to figure out what really mattered. I had to become someone I could be proud of. Someone they could be proud of, too."

That night, after the last balloon had floated away and Emma and Lucas had gone home with Jake and Rebecca, Mark and I walked through the park together. The same path we'd walked two years earlier when we first met. Me still cautious, him quietly steady.

We stopped near the lake, the water catching the gold of the setting sun. Ducks drifted along the surface, and the air had that peaceful hush that only comes at the end of a full, happy day.

"I have something to ask you," Mark said, suddenly a little nervous.

I turned to him. "Okay..."

He reached into his jacket pocket and pulled out a small velvet box, then got down on one knee. The moment stretched, soft and full of breath.

"Emily," he said, looking up at me with eyes full of steady love, "will you marry me?"

I stared at him. This man who had held space for my healing, who never tried to fix me, just stood beside me as I learned how to fix myself. This man who'd earned Emma and Lucas's trust one quiet moment at a time.

"Yes," I said, tears already streaming down my cheeks. "Yes. Absolutely, yes."

The ring was simple and perfect, like everything that mattered. When he slipped it onto my finger and pulled me into a hug, I felt something click into place not because he completed me, but because I'd finally grown whole enough to love and be loved, fully and honestly.

"Have you talked to Emma and Lucas?" I asked, wiping tears from my face.

"I asked them last week," he said. "Emma wanted to know if she could help plan the wedding. Lucas wanted to make sure I'd still help him with his science projects."

"And what did you say?"

"I told Emma she's in charge of flowers," Mark said with a smile. "And I told Lucas I'm not going anywhere."

We stood there a long while, watching the ducks, holding hands, breathing in the quiet. It wasn't the life I'd planned, but it was the one I'd earned.

And it was enough. More than enough.

Six months later, I stood in the tiny bridal room of the chapel Mark and I had chosen for our wedding, staring into the mirror like I was trying to memorize the woman in front of me. I wore a soft blue dress, nothing extravagant, nothing white. This wasn't my first wedding, and blue had always been Mark's favorite color. More than that, it made me feel beautiful. Not flashy or disguised, just me at peace in my own skin.

I didn't rush. I just looked.

The last time I'd really looked at myself, really studied the person in the mirror, had been over three years earlier. That night in my apartment, after the police had left, after they'd asked to see my children, after I'd stood at the edge of losing everything. I remembered that version of me: eyes rimmed red from too much wine and too little sleep, cheeks sunken, skin dull and sallow. A kind of tired that sleep couldn't fix. A kind of despair that settled in the bones.

The woman in front of me now looked different. Not younger. Not flawless. But alive.

My eyes were clear. My cheeks had color. My smile, when it appeared, without effort lit up my whole face. There were faint laugh lines around my eyes now, the kind you earn from joy, not pain. My hair was pinned simply but neatly. I looked like a woman who belonged to her own life.

And I whispered it, soft and amazed, "Happy Mommy..."

Emma had drawn that picture years ago, back when I didn't deserve the title but clung to it anyway. Now, finally, I wasn't just pretending to be her. I was her.

This was the woman Mark had fallen in love with. This was the mother Emma and Lucas trusted again. This was who I had fought, every single day, to become. Not some polished version of perfection, but someone whole. Someone real. Someone sober and grounded and here.

I lifted a hand to the mirror with my fingertips brushing the glass. It felt like reaching for an old friend I thought I'd lost for good.

"Thank you," I whispered to the woman looking back at me. "Thank you for holding on."

A single tear slid down my cheek, warm against skin that finally looked alive again.

Emma knocked gently on the door, dressed in the pale yellow dress she'd picked out as my maid of honor.

"Are you ready?" she asked.

"I think so. Are you ready to help me walk down the aisle?"

"Yes. Lucas is ready too. He's been practicing with the rings all morning."

We'd decided that instead of my father giving me away, Emma and Lucas would walk me down the aisle. A symbol that this marriage was about joining families, not just two people.

The ceremony was small, just fifty people who had been part of our recovery and rebuilding. Linda was there, beaming. My parents cried openly. Jake and Rebecca stood together, hands clasped, the final sign of our blended family's healing.

When the minister asked who supported this union, the entire congregation stood up.

As Mark and I exchanged the vows we'd written ourselves, I looked out at the faces of everyone who had witnessed my journey back from rock bottom.

"I promise to love you not because I need you," I said, "but because I choose you. I promise to be present for our joys and our challenges. I promise never to escape from our life together with anything other than honesty and breath. And I promise to love your stepchildren as carefully as you love mine."

Mark smiled and took my hands. "I promise to love you exactly as you are, and to support who you're becoming. I promise to be patient when recovery is hard, and to celebrate every milestone with you. I promise to love Emma and Lucas as if they were my own, while always respecting the wonderful father they already have."

When the minister pronounced us husband and wife, Emma and Lucas cheered louder than anyone.

At the reception, held in the same community center where I now ran my Thursday night support group, Jake raised a toast.

"To Emily and Mark," he said, holding up his glass, "who prove that families can be rebuilt with love, patience, and forgiveness. And to Emma and Lucas, who are getting another adult who loves them unconditionally."

Later that night, after we'd hugged the last guest goodbye, Mark and I tucked the kids into their new bedrooms in our small, sunlit three-bedroom house. Everyone had their own space now, but we were all together.

"Are you happy, Mommy?" Emma asked as I kissed her forehead.

"So happy," I said. "Are you?"

"Yes. I like this story better than the old one."

"Me too, sweetheart. Me too."

After the kids were asleep, Mark and I sat on the back porch, wrapped in a blanket, sipping herbal tea under the stars.

"Any regrets?" he asked.

I thought about it. About the affair that detonated my first marriage. The wine I chose over everything. The night in the hospital bed with my mother clutching my hand. The custody loss. The supervised visits. The shame. The fight. The climb.

"No," I said finally. "Not anymore. All of that brought me here. To this version of myself. I wouldn't change any of it because changing it might mean I never became someone worthy of this life."

Mark reached for my hand. I looked down at my wedding ring, resting beside the three-year sobriety chip I still kept in my pocket like a talisman.

"You know what I learned in recovery?" I said.

"What?"

"That rock bottom isn't the end of your story. It's the foundation you build your real life on."

Above us, the stars stretched wide and bright, quiet witnesses to the long road back.

Tomorrow would bring what it always brings. Work emails, parenting decisions, moments of fear, moments of grace. The daily, beautiful maintenance of love and sobriety and a life earned.

But tonight, I was exactly where I belonged. Not because I'd gotten my old life back, but because I'd built a new one.

A life grounded in truth, not shame. In presence, not escape. In love, not need.

A life where Happy Mommy wasn't just a mask I put on during visits, but who I truly was.

A life worth staying sober for.

One day at a time. Forever.

Chapter Thirteen

Bonus: The Sober Toolkit That Actually Works

THANK YOU FOR READING this far. Making it to the end of this book means you're serious about change or at least open to seeing what a different path could look like. I'm grateful you've spent your time with these stories, and I hope some of what you've read here has made your own journey feel a little less lonely.

I know how challenging it can be to face real-life situations where cravings sneak up or old habits call your name. That's exactly why I created the Sober Toolkit, a collection of practical strategies, quick reminders, and real-world tips you can turn to when you need something that works in the moment. These are the same tools I've leaned on myself, and they've helped not just me but many others stay steady and keep moving forward.

If you want an extra boost, some honest encouragement, or just a practical game plan for the next tough event, I'd love for you to check out the toolkit. Use the link or QR code below to visit the website, where you can download the toolkit document. It's my way of saying thank you for reading, and of sharing something that's helped me and so many others. Whether you're at day one or year five, the toolkit is there for you whenever you need it—and you might be surprised by how much a simple idea or new approach can help right when you need it most.

Link to the Sober Toolkit

https://selfcarejourneybooks.com/books/from-wine-mom-to-sober-mom/

Chapter Fourteen

Bonus: The Double Life of a High-Functioning Alcoholic

If you're looking for more inspiration on the path to sobriety, I've included the first section of my other alcohol recovery story book, *The Double Life of a High-Functioning Alcoholic*, just below. It's a raw and honest look at what happens when drinking hides behind success and what it takes to finally break free.

Invisible Line

I wasn't the kind of guy who was supposed to have a drinking problem.

That thought pulsed through my head as I stared into the hotel bathroom mirror, clutching the sink like it might steady the panic in my chest. The place was high-end. Sleek marble, soft lighting, one of those fancy hotels in Manhattan where the soap smells like eucalyptus. We were there for my company's big data science summit. I was supposed to be the calm, collected director, the guy running a global team, presenting on machine learning pipelines, shaking hands with VPs.

Instead, I was hiding.

My hands trembled just enough to betray me. Not so anyone would notice. I'd become too good at that. I kept them under the table during meetings, wrapped around a mug of black coffee like it was armor, or buried deep in my blazer pockets while I gave polished presentations.

"Everything okay in there, Dave?" my VP called through the door.

I flinched.

"Yep! All good. Be right out," I said, way too casually.

I turned on the tap and let the cold water run over my wrists. That trick had worked before. I took a few deep breaths, stared at myself in the mirror, and straightened my tie. When I walked back out into the ballroom, I looked like I had it all together.

No one could tell I'd blacked out the night before. Again.

No one knew I'd woken up at 3 a.m. with my heart pounding, scrolling through texts, trying to piece together what I'd said to my team at the happy hour. Or whether I'd embarrassed myself. Again.

I was forty-four. Married, with a son who thought I hung the moon. From the outside, things looked great. I had a career most people would kill for, leading a team of twenty data scientists spread across three continents. I could talk about neural nets and predictive models like I was reciting the alphabet.

And I could also outdrink a room full of consultants, then be up at six the next morning for a client call like nothing happened.

From the outside, I was the furthest thing from an "alcoholic." I didn't drink in the mornings. Never touched vodka in the garage. I could go a week (sometimes two) without a drop. I just liked to "unwind." You know, the way a lot of high-performing, over-caffeinated professionals do. The problem was, "unwind" had quietly morphed into "unravel."

The cracks were small at first. A foggy memory here. A missed bedtime story there. A few too many on a Thursday night that turned into an argument with my wife over nothing.

But that day in the hotel bathroom, something shifted. I couldn't ignore the signs anymore. My body was jittery. My mind was racing. And underneath the mask of composure, I felt like a guy dangling from a cliff edge, pretending he was just out for a scenic hike.

I once read that the most dangerous part of drinking isn't going from sober to drunk. It's crossing that invisible line between drinking in control and drinking that quietly controls you. The catch is, you don't notice when you've crossed it. You just wake up one day and realize the line's behind you.

This isn't a story about a dramatic rock bottom. I didn't crash my car. I didn't lose my job or get arrested. My life, from the outside, still looked perfectly intact. But inside, I was slowly unraveling.

And that's the thing no one tells you. Alcohol doesn't have to wreck your life overnight to be a problem. Sometimes, it erodes you in tiny, invisible ways. It chips away at your clarity, your confidence, your peace of mind. It steals the little moments: the bedtime stories, the weekend mornings, the honest conversations. And you don't even realize how much you've lost until you try to stop.

This memoir isn't about rock bottom. It's about the gray area where everything still looks okay, but nothing feels right. It's about the long, messy decision to quit drinking when everyone around you says, "But you don't have a problem." It's about making that decision, anyway.

It's also about what happens next. Because quitting isn't some magical fix. It's not an overnight glow-up. It's a quiet revolution.

One day at a time, one awkward social event at a time, one lonely Friday night at a time. You trade numbness for clarity, which sounds great until you remember how much easier life was to ignore when you were a little buzzed.

But here's the thing. Clarity, even when it hurts, is worth it.

My story doesn't begin with disaster. It begins with a mirror, a pair of shaking hands, and a man realizing that something has to change. It begins in that foggy, familiar space between "I'm fine" and "I'm not." And maybe that's where your story begins too.

If you've ever looked at your life and thought, This looks great on paper, so why do I feel like I'm falling apart? This is for you.

If you've ever asked yourself, Do I really need to stop? Even as some small, honest part of you whispers, Maybe you do. Then yeah, this is definitely for you.

It's for all of us who weren't "supposed" to have a problem, but found ourselves face-to-face with one, anyway.

The First Taste

Sitting on the cold bathroom floor of that Manhattan hotel, hands still shaking, I kept circling back to one question: How did I end up here? When did drinking for fun turn into drinking just to function? There was no dramatic moment that marked the change. The story really started over twenty years earlier with a simple invitation and a lie I told myself about being able to handle anything that came my way.

Senior year of high school, 1998. I was seventeen and every little thing seemed to carry life-or-death importance. Katie Morrison stood at her locker, talking to Jake Stevens about the weekend. Jake was everything I wanted to be: confident, relaxed, the kind of guy who could fit in anywhere.

I hung around, pretending to search my backpack while I listened in.

"My parents are going to my aunt's wedding this weekend," Katie said. "You guys should come over Saturday night."

My heart was pounding. Katie was throwing a party. This was the same Katie I had a crush on since tenth grade, but never had the guts to ask out.

I told myself this was my chance. Every movie I watched said all I needed was the courage to speak up. If I was honest, I could win her over.

My legs felt heavy as I forced myself to walk over. My mouth was dry, but in my head I could hear my father saying, "Dave, you're just as smart as those kids."

I took a shaky breath and joined the conversation.

"Hey, Katie," I said, voice a little thin. "Um, your party sounds fun. Is it okay if I come?"

She turned, smiling in that way she always did. "Of course, Dave. You should come."

I almost asked her to say it again, just to make sure I heard right. Katie Morrison had just invited me to her party.

The rest of that week, I was caught somewhere between excitement and panic. My best friend, Marcus Chen, tried to bring me down to earth.

"You know there's going to be drinking, right?" he asked at lunch.

"So?" I replied, already searching the internet for 'how to be cool at parties.'

"You've never even had a drink before."

He was right. My family had a long history of alcohol problems, and my parents always warned me to be careful. They talked about addiction like it was a shadow that could fall over anyone if you were not paying attention.

"It's not about the drinking," I told Marcus. "It's about finally feeling like I belong."

By Saturday night, I had convinced myself this party would change everything. Maybe after this, I would stop being invisible.

Katie's house was in one of those perfect suburban neighborhoods where every yard looked manicured and every porch light was on. I parked three blocks away, partly because the street was full, but mostly because I didn't want anyone to see our old, dented Honda Civic.

As I walked up to the door, I could hear music and laughter spilling out onto the lawn. I rang the bell and rehearsed something clever to say.

Katie answered, casually in jeans and a sweater. "Dave! You made it!"

I followed her inside. The living room was filled with twenty or so kids from our class. This wasn't the wild party from the movies. It felt more grown-up, which somehow made me even more aware of my khakis and button-down shirt.

I found my way to the snack table and loaded up on chips, pretending I knew what I was doing. I watched the room and tried to work up the nerve to talk to anyone. Jake was at the center of it all, making everyone laugh.

I was thinking about making up an excuse to leave when Jake looked over and spotted me.

"Hey, brain boy! Glad you made it," he called out, waving me over.

To my surprise, he seemed genuinely happy I was there. He even moved over on the couch to make space for me.

"Davies, you look like you're about to have a panic attack," he teased, grinning.

He was not wrong. My shoulders were tense and my smile felt forced. I probably looked like I was about to bolt for the door.

That was the moment Jake reached into a cooler and pulled out a beer.

The can in Jake's hand was ice-cold, little drops of condensation forming on the outside. He held it out to me, casual as ever, like passing a drink was just the most natural thing to do.

"This will help you loosen up, man."

I stared at the beer as if it might explode. In seventeen years, nobody my age had ever offered me alcohol.

"I don't really drink," I said, which was the understatement of my life.

Jake grinned and shrugged off my hesitation. "That's even better. Tonight is your big initiation. Welcome to the real world, Davies."

The real world. Sometimes it felt like my parents' warnings about alcohol had just kept me on the outside of everything. Maybe there was something here I was supposed to learn about being normal.

I looked around. Everyone had a drink. Beer cans, red cups. Even Marcus, who had warned me about this, stood by the fireplace with a beer in his hand, deep in conversation.

Jake leaned in a little closer. "You're smart, Davies, but you overthink everything. Sometimes you have to just trust yourself."

That sounded like advice for a science test, but maybe it applied here too.

I took the beer from him. It felt heavy and colder than I expected, almost numbing my hand. I pulled the tab, and the sharp hiss made a few people glance over. Suddenly, I felt very exposed.

The smell was nothing like I expected. Sharp and yeasty, not at all like anything I thought grown-up drinks should smell like. I hesitated, then raised the can and took my first sip.

The taste was terrible. Bitter, harsh, nothing pleasant about it. I wanted to set the can down and forget the whole thing, but I could feel eyes on me. Katie had wandered over to our group and seemed curious to see what I would do.

I swallowed and tried not to let my face show how bad it was.

"Not bad, right?" Jake said.

I nodded, not trusting myself to speak. Still, I noticed something changing almost right away. A warm feeling started in my chest, a little bubble of relaxation that felt new and strangely welcome.

Katie took a seat across from us. "How do you feel?"

"Good," I answered, surprised by how easy my voice sounded. "Different, but good."

She smiled. "Different how?"

I took another sip, focusing on the feeling more than the taste this time. The warmth kept spreading, and the room seemed to soften around the edges. Conversations were easier to follow. My anxiety felt lighter.

"It's like everything isn't so intense," I said.

Jake clinked his can against mine. "Welcome to the club, Davies."

The second sip was easier. After half the can, I noticed the people around me started to make more sense. I was no longer over-analyzing every word, every look. I was just there, listening.

Jake launched into a story about last weekend's football game. Normally, I would have been in my head, worrying about how to respond. This time, I just listened and when he mentioned calling an audible, I found myself asking, "What's that?"

"It means changing the play at the last minute," Jake said. "Sometimes you have to go with your gut instead of the plan."

That sounded familiar. I shared how my best SAT scores came from trusting my first instinct.

Katie leaned in, interested. "What did you get?"

"Fifteen eighty," I answered, and then worried I sounded full of myself.

Jake let out a low whistle. "That's incredible, Davies."

"Amazing," Katie said, and the warmth inside me grew. For a moment, I was just happy. No calculations, no rehearsing what to say next.

I kept talking, words coming easily now. "The stress was the worst part. I kept thinking about how much was riding on that test."

Sarah Martinez, who I barely knew, joined in. "I hate that pressure. Why should four hours on a Saturday decide your entire future?"

I agreed. "The sections I stressed over most were my lowest scores. Anxiety just makes you dumber."

Everyone nodded. I took another sip, barely noticing the taste. Everything felt easier.

For the first time, I felt like I finally fit in. For a little while, I felt normal.

Jake handed me a second beer without saying a word. This time, I did not hesitate. The taste was already less harsh, almost neutral now. What mattered more was how my mind felt. I was not slower, just less cluttered. Everything seemed easier.

"So what's MIT going to be like?" Sarah asked as she sat down next to me on the couch.

Sarah Martinez was talking to me by choice. Three hours ago, I would have been too anxious to get a sentence out.

"Hopefully like this," I said, motioning around the room, "but with a lot more calculus."

Everyone laughed, and it was genuine laughter, not just polite agreement.

"You're way funnier than I thought," Katie said, and I felt a different kind of warmth, one that had nothing to do with alcohol.

Way funnier than she thought. That meant she had thought about me before. I had never considered that.

I was getting the hang of this, whatever this was. Making conversation, being part of things, just showing up as myself. And the beer seemed to be the key. Not drinking to get drunk, but finding just the right amount, so my usual anxiety dropped away and my personality could actually come through.

"The real problem with high school," I said, ideas coming out fast and easy, "is that everyone is pretending to be someone they're not. We're all acting out these roles we think we're supposed to play."

Katie nodded like she understood. "Yes. Like, I'm supposed to be the perfect student government president, but half the time I have no clue what I'm doing."

"You seem pretty natural at it," I said.

"That's just because I'm getting better at faking confidence," she admitted. "Inside, I'm terrified I'm about to mess everything up."

I stared at her. Katie, nervous about screwing up? The same girl who could give speeches to the entire school?

"Everyone's got their own stuff going on," Jake said. "The trick is not letting it show."

But why should we all have to hide our nerves? The alcohol was giving me a new way to look at the connection. I started to see that real relationships were built on letting some of that fear show.

Suddenly everyone was sharing these honest moments I had always thought were just mine. The beer was not just making me more social. It was making all of us more open.

I reached for my third beer without thinking about it. My hand just knew what to do.

"Look at Davies. Go," Jake said, giving me an approving nod.

Something was shifting inside me. The anxious, overthinking version of myself was still there, but now he was in the background. Out front was someone who could tell a story, make people laugh, and even get attention from Katie.

Katie kept glancing my way. For the first time, I believed I might actually have a chance with her.

The third beer was easier to drink than the first two. Now the edges of the world felt soft and easy. I found myself telling a story about my physics teacher when Jake put his hand on my shoulder.

"Easy, champ. Maybe slow down."

I looked down and realized I already had a fourth beer in my hand. I did not even remember opening it.

"I'm fine," I said, and I meant it. I felt better than fine. I felt like I was finally winning at something that used to defeat me.

Slowing down did not make sense. Why would I stop when everything was going so well? People were laughing. I was being included, and Katie had already asked me three questions about college. It felt like this was what I had been missing all along.

I finished my fourth beer and immediately felt the absence of it. I wanted to hold on to this feeling a little longer.

"I should get another," I said.

"Maybe take a break?" Marcus suggested, but his voice felt far away.

A break from confidence and being included? That felt like the exact wrong move.

I made my way back to the cooler, weaving around groups. As I reached in for another beer, I caught a glimpse of myself in the window. For a moment, I hardly recognized the person looking back. I looked relaxed, smiling easily, moving like I belonged at parties.

I grabbed a fifth beer and walked back, floating on air.

The fifth beer felt like a victory. It seemed like I had finally found the answer to every social problem I ever had. Katie was talking about the stress of college applications, and I nodded along, convinced I understood everything.

"The worst part is writing those essays," she said. "How do you sum up your whole life in just a few hundred words?"

"You pick a single moment that stands for it all," I said, leaning in. "Like this party."

Jake grinned. "This party is your entire life now?"

"This party is when I stopped sitting on the sidelines and started living," I replied. I thought I sounded poetic.

Katie looked at me with something close to admiration. "That's actually beautiful, Dave."

Her words gave me a rush. Suddenly, I wanted to say everything I'd ever felt.

"Katie," I blurted out, "I need to tell you something."

The room faded into the background. I felt like it was just us.

"I've had feelings for you since sophomore year," I said. "You're not just beautiful. You're kind, and smart, and you make everyone feel important."

The words spilled out. In my mind, this kind of honesty had to be right.

Katie's expression changed, but in my beer-fueled state, I thought it meant she was moved. She just looked surprised.

"Dave, you're really drunk right now," she said softly.

Drunk? I shook my head. I was just being honest for once.

"I'm not drunk. I'm telling the truth. I love you. I've loved you for years."

But Katie pulled back, and Jake stood up. I suddenly felt everyone in the room watching us. The laughter and music died down.

"Katie, please," I said, my voice rising. "I know you feel something, too. We have a connection."

Jake stepped in. "Dave, you need to stop."

Stop? I could not stop now. I was so close to finally saying everything.

"I love you," I said, my words echoing in the now-quiet room.

The silence was crushing. Katie's face turned pale, and not in a good way. I realized too late she felt only discomfort and pity.

"Oh, Dave," she said quietly. "You're really drunk. This isn't how this works."

Her words cut through me. I looked around. Every face showed the same thing: embarrassment for me.

"Katie, I—" I started, but Jake gently stepped between us.

"Come on, buddy. Let's get you some water."

I tried to push past him. "Don't call me buddy. This is between me and Katie."

At that moment, I lost my balance and stumbled. It was not a dramatic fall, but it might as well have been.

The spell was broken. People started talking again, quieter this time, and I heard the laughter behind me.

Jake took my arm. "Let's get some water."

I let him lead me to the kitchen, but I kept looking back at Katie, hoping she might understand.

Instead, she was talking to Sarah, both of them looking worried and a little scared.

That was when it hit me. I had ruined everything.

The Rest of Chapters...

Find the complete story and more alcohol recovery books by Howard Kane on Amazon. Scan the code or copy the link into your browser to start reading. Available in Paperback, Kindle, Kindle Unlimited, and Audiobook.

Link to Amazon Alcohol Recovery Book Series

https://www.amazon.com/dp/B0FNDHYW58

This page was intentionally left blank.

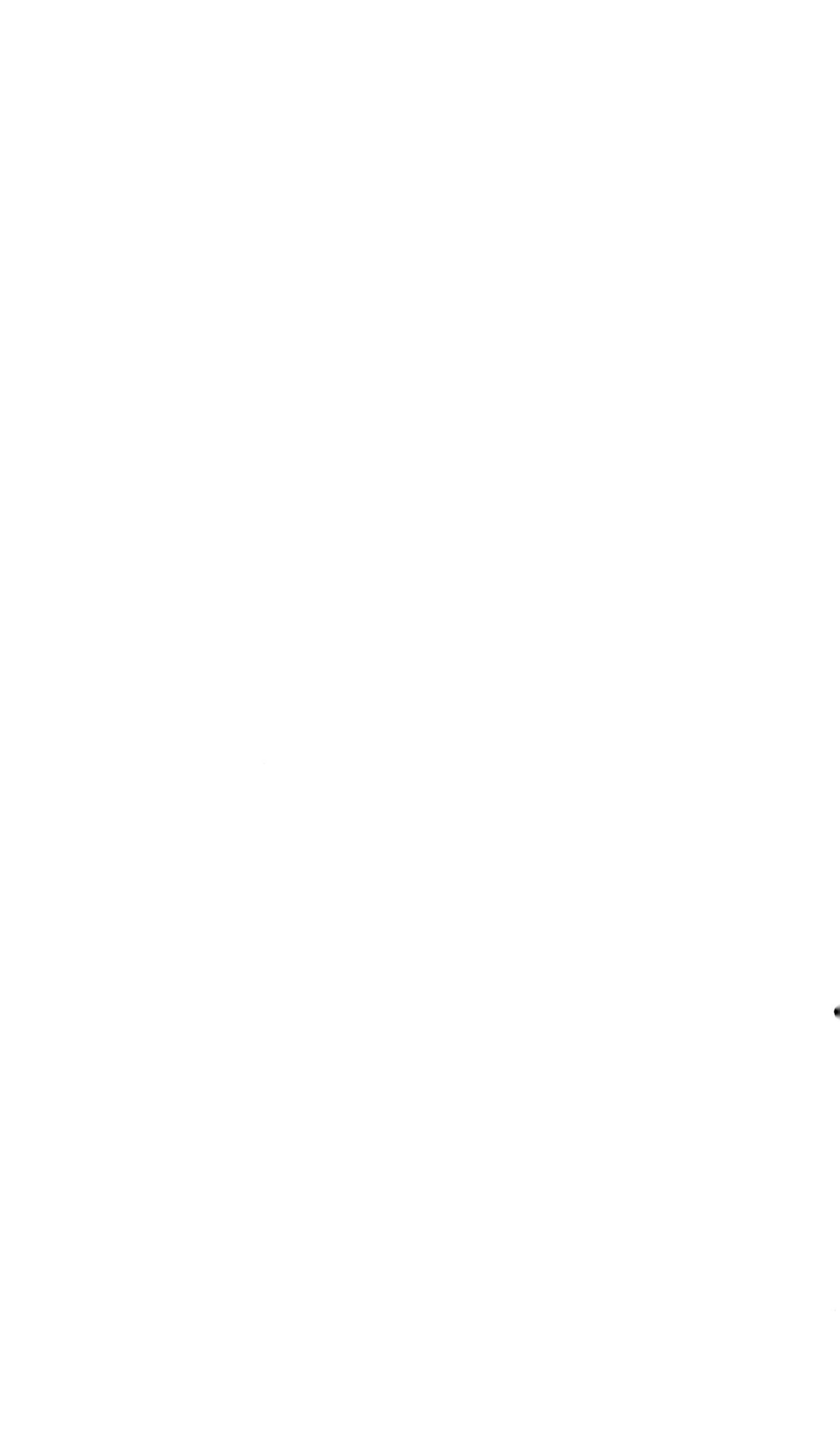

www.ingramcontent.com/pod-product-compliance
Lightning Source LLC
Chambersburg PA
CBHW070106030426
42335CB00016B/2027